Meniscal Injuries

John D. Kelly IV

Editor

Meniscal Injuries

Management and Surgical Techniques

Springer

2014

Editor
John D. Kelly IV, M.D.
Associate Professor of Orthopedic Surgery
Hospital of the University of Pennsylvania
Philadelphia, PA, USA

ISBN 978-1-4614-8485-1   ISBN 978-1-4614-8486-8 (eBook)
DOI 10.1007/978-1-4614-8486-8
Springer New York Heidelberg Dordrecht London

Library of Congress Control Number: 2013948916

Printed on acid-free paper

Springer is part of Springer Science+Business Media (www.springer.com)

I dedicate this book to the woman of my dreams, the answer to my prayers, my best friend and soul mate and ticket to heaven—my lovely wife of 25 years, Marie Therese Sakosky Kelly. Marie has been a source of loving kindness and support throughout my professional life. She has raised two exceptional daughters, Ann Marie and Mary Elizabeth, and has endured the countless "call nights," "add on cases," emergencies, and demands of a busy surgical practice with grace and understanding. She has simply afforded me the opportunity to fulfill my professional dreams.

Foreword

It is timely and important to devote a comprehensive book entirely to knee meniscus surgery. This multiauthored book has been carefully conceived, edited, and partially authored by John D. Kelly IV, M.D. He and his contributing authors have captured the breathtaking growth in appreciation and understanding of the important roles that the menisci play in the overall health and function of the knee, and the continuing evolution of surgical procedures to address meniscus injuries while preserving as much functional meniscus tissue as possible, over the relatively short span of the past 40 years. This book is rich with principles, guidelines, and in-depth details of diagnosis of meniscus injuries, decision making, surgical techniques, aftercare (including rehabilitation), and current outcomes and updates of clinical and basic science research aimed at enhancing meniscus repair, regeneration, and replacement. It is also well illustrated and referenced.

Interested readers will appreciate the scholarly review of the essential foundation information contained in the first three chapters that cover meniscal anatomy, patient history, and physical examination, including an in-depth description of the many clinical tests to evaluate the menisci (including one that was new to me—the Thessaly test), and imaging of meniscus pathology. A group of six chapters address surgical treatment: partial meniscectomy, indications for meniscus repair, repair techniques with a separate chapter for diagnosis and repair of meniscal root avulsion, meniscus allograft transplantation, and rehabilitation following meniscus repair. The remaining three chapters address ongoing exciting basic science research focused on developing and testing of differing approaches to improve meniscus healing and/or regeneration: meniscus scaffolds, enhancement of repair, and biological augmentation of meniscus repair and restoration.

I recommend this book highly and encourage any orthopaedic surgeon who is interested in arthroscopic knee surgery to not only obtain a copy but also read it carefully. No matter how experienced or inexperienced you may be, there is much to learn from what I expect to become a major resource in this area for a long time to come.

Rochester, NY, USA   Kenneth E. DeHaven, M.D.

Preface

Meniscal injuries are clearly the most common affliction a knee surgeon will encounter. Indeed, the diagnosis and treatment of meniscal tears are the "life-blood" of a sports medicine practice. Once regarded as a "vestigial" structure, the role of the meniscus as crucial element of knee function and health has never been more evident. With increasing longevity and active lifestyles of aging patients, the preservation of meniscal integrity has become increasingly important.

This book endeavors to enlighten the reader with recent scientific data which will assist in the timely recognition and treatment of meniscal lesions. It is my sincere hope and expectation that this book will convey to health care practitioners evidence-based "pearls" which will translate to improved patient care and meniscal preservation.

I am indebted to my authors—all thought leaders in meniscus science. Their contributions have helped create this treatise on the most recent scientific developments pertaining to meniscal function, mechanics, replacement, imaging, diagnosis, surgical repair, and rehabilitation.

I wish to thank the "forefathers" of meniscal surgery—such visionaries as Drs. Ken DeHaven, Dilworth Cannon, and Charles Henning who recognized the value of meniscal repair when contemporaries considered the meniscus as a dispensable structure.

I am indebted to my teachers, Drs. Joseph Torg, James Nixon, and John Lachman, who taught me timeless principles of caring for patients with musculoskeletal injuries. I am especially grateful for the blessing of an exceptional mentor, Ray A. Moyer M.D., who taught me innumerable lessons in patient care, and, more importantly, in integrity, honesty, and conservative treatment. The wisdom I gained under Dr. Moyer's tutelage continues to serve my patients well. I steadfastly share Dr. Moyer's instruction on ethically based and compassionate care to medical students, residents, and fellows at every opportunity.

I wish to acknowledge my Chairman, L. Scott Levin, M.D., who has supported my academic interests and has nurtured a unique culture of scientific investigation and discovery at the department of Orthopedic Surgery at the University of Penn. In addition, my colleague and Chief of Sports Medicine, Brian Sennett, M.D., has indeed been the "partner from heaven" in that he has wholeheartedly supported my educational, research, and clinical interests from the moment I joined Penn 5 years ago.

Jennifer Schneider, developmental editor, has been a positive and encouraging force who has demonstrated exceptional patience and kindness to both me and the other authors. I truly appreciate her professionalism, expertise, and skill, all clothed in courtesy.

Finally, I wish to thank my family, who, next to my faith, has been the singular most important source of energy in my life. My parents, John D. and Loretta T. Kelly, made innumerable sacrifices to finance my education and instructed me well in "old world" values. I have the gifts of a sister, Mary Ann, who is fiercely loyal and loving and a twin brother, Michael, who has "covered my back" his entire lifetime.

My daughters, Mary and Ann Marie, have brought me more joy than any parent could imagine. I marvel how they have blossomed into intelligent and service-oriented young women. My wife of 25 years, Marie, who I fondly refer to as "Santa Maria," has been a continual source of love, loyalty, and wisdom. Her unconditional support, through "thick and thin," continually energizes me so that my dreams, such as this book, can be realized.

Philadelphia, PA, USA   John D. Kelly IV, M.D.

Contents

Contributors

Geoffrey D. Abrams, M.D. Department of Orthopedic Surgery, Rush University Medical Center, Chicago, IL, USA

Nicole S. Belkin, M.D. Department of Orthopaedic Surgery, Hospital of the University of Pennsylvania, Philadelphia, PA, USA

James L. Carey, M.D., M.P.H. Department of Orthopaedic Surgery, Penn Center for Advanced Cartilage Repair and Osteochondritis Dissecans Treatment, Hospital of the University of Pennsylvania, Philadelphia, PA, USA

Brian J. Cole, M.D., M.B.A. Department of Orthopedic Surgery, Rush University Medical Center, Chicago, IL, USA

Brian Eckenrode, P.T., D.P.T., O.C.S. Department of Physical Therapy, Arcadia University, Glenside, PA, USA

Matthew B. Fisher, Ph.D. Department of Orthopaedic Surgery, University of Pennsylvania, Philadelphia, PA, USA

Anil K. Gupta, M.D., M.B.A. Department of Orthopedic Surgery, Rush University Medical Center, Chicago, IL, USA

Joshua D. Harris, M.D. Department of Orthopedic Surgery, Rush University Medical Center, Chicago, IL, USA

John G. Horneff III, M.D. Department of Orthopaedic Surgery, Hospital of the University of Pennsylvania, Philadelphia, PA, USA

Jason E. Hsu, M.D. Department of Orthopaedic Surgery, Hospital of the University of Pennsylvania, Philadelphia, PA, USA

Ann Marie Kelly Department of Orthopedics, University of Pennsylvania, Philadelphia, PA, USA

John D. Kelly IV, M.D. Department of Orthopaedic Surgery, Hospital of the University of Pennsylvania, Philadelphia, PA, USA

Viviane Khoury, M.D. Department of Radiology, University of Pennsylvania, Philadelphia, PA, USA

Peter R. Kurzweil, M.D. Memorial Orthopaedic Surgical Group, Long Beach, CA, USA

Robert L. Mauck, Ph.D. Mckay Orthopaedic Research Laboratory, University of Pennsylvania, Philadelphia, PA, USA

Frank A. McCormick, M.D. Department of Orthopedic Surgery, Rush University Medical Center, Chicago, IL, USA

Kevin J. McHale, M.D. Department of Orthopaedic Surgery, Hospital of the University of Pennsylvania, Philadelphia, PA, USA

Min Jung Park, M.D., M.M.Sc. Department of Orthopaedic Surgery, Hospital of the University of Pennsylvania, Philadelphia, PA, USA

Christos D. Photopoulos, M.D. Hospital of the University of Pennsylvania, Philadelphia, PA, USA

Marisa Pontillo, P.T., D.P.T., S.C.S. GSPP Penn Therapy and Fitness at Penn Sports Medicine Center, Philadelphia, PA, USA

Feini Qu, B.S.E. Department of Orthopaedic Surgery, University of Pennsylvania, Philadelphia, PA, USA

Brian J. Sennett, M.D. Department of Orthopaedic Surgery, Penn Sports Medicine Center, University of Pennsylvania, Philadelphia, PA, USA

Amy E. Sewick, M.D. Department of Orthopaedic Surgery, Hospital of the University of Pennsylvania, Philadelphia, PA, USA

K. Donald Shelbourne, M.D. Shelbourne Knee Center, Indianapolis, IN, USA

Fotios Paul Tjoumakaris, M.D. Department of Orthopaedic Surgery, Jefferson Medical College, Rothman Institute Orthopaedics, Egg Harbor Township, NJ, USA

Stephen J. Torres, M.D., B.S. Department of Orthopaedic Surgery, Hospital of the University of Pennsylvania, Philadelphia, PA, USA

Scott E. Urch, M.D. Shelbourne Knee Center, Indianapolis, IN, USA

Pramod B. Voleti, M.D. Department of Orthopaedic Surgery, Hospital of the University of Pennsylvania, Philadelphia, PA, USA

Meniscal Anatomy

Stephen J. Torres, Jason E. Hsu,
and Robert L. Mauck

Introduction

The word meniscus derives from the Greek word *meniskos* which means crescent. There are a number of menisci through the human body, including in the temporomandibular joint, the sternoclavicular joint, the acromioclavicular joint, and the knee joint. The largest of these menisci are the two located in the knee joint, which are named for their position: the medial meniscus and lateral meniscus. The focus of this chapter will be the structure of the meniscus and the anatomical features that are important to the function of the knee joint. Also important will be how those features are implicated in injuries of the meniscus and the principles that govern the treatment of meniscal pathology. While previously thought to be useless "remnants of muscle within the knee joint," the menisci play important roles in the knee joint and their anatomical features are distinctly unique and afford their myriad functions.

S.J. Torres, M.D., B.S. (✉) • J.E. Hsu, M.D.
Department of Orthopaedic Surgery, Hospital of
the University of Pennsylvania, 3400 Spruce Street,
2 Silverstein, Philadelphia, PA 19104, USA
e-mail: Stephen.torres@uphs.upenn.edu

R.L. Mauck, Ph.D.
Mckay Orthopaedic Research Laboratory, University
of Pennsylvania, Philadelphia, PA 19104, USA

Embryonic Development

In early embryonic development the lower limb buds first appear around 4 weeks after fertilization [1]. At 6 weeks, the femur, tibia, and fibula begin to undergo chondrification and a distinct joint is seen around 7 weeks, as depicted by an undifferentiated blastemal zone between the femur and tibia. By 7½ weeks the blastema organizes into three distinct layers. By 8 weeks, the menisci become distinct structures and are formed from mesenchymal cells that originate from the intermediate layer of the chondrogenic blastema. Recent lineage tracing studies suggest that these cells arise from both the surrounding perichondrium and from the cartilage anlagen itself [2]. During weeks 8–16, the joint cavity continues to develop, forming the basis of the articulating knee joint [1, 3, 4]. From a developmental standpoint, the meniscus already possesses a distinct alignment of cells and nascent extracellular matrix early in gestation. With maturation and further development, the cell number decreases while the aligned collagenous matrix becomes increasingly dominant [5]. As this extracellular matrix matures, the tissue becomes increasingly less vascularized, such that in the adult, vascularity supplies only the outer ~25 % nearest the synovial margins.

Histology

The functional cell types seen with in the adult meniscus are primarily fibrochondrocytes. The outer two-thirds of the meniscus has an appearance similar to fibrocartilage, whereas the inner one-third is more resembling of hyaline cartilage [6–8]. There have been four distinct varieties of fibrochondrocytes cells described, depending on their position within the architecture of the meniscus. The superficial portion of the meniscus has fusiform cells similar in appearance to flattened chondrocytes that contain long cytoplasmic projections which form a complex network with adjacent cells [9, 10]. The deeper cells are typically ovoid in shape and have an appearance similar to chondrocytes of the transitional and radial zones of the articular cartilage [10]. These cells have no direct contact and are evenly distributed throughout the extracellular matrix. Dispersed between these two regions are two additional cell types that differ only in the number of cytoplasmic projections [9]. This orientation is important in forming the framework of the meniscus.

The fibrocartilaginous architecture of the meniscus plays an important role in its overall function and, through scanning electron microscopy, can be divided into three layers (see Fig. 1.1). The superficial layers consist of fine collagen fibrils arranged parallel to the surface in a mesh-like pattern. Deep to this are larger collagen fibers oriented in a radial direction with intersecting fibers of varying angles dispersed throughout. The deep layer constitutes the bulk of the meniscus; these fibers are oriented in a circumferential fashion [11–13]. This orientation is important in giving the meniscus its biomechanical strength which is highest in tension in the circumferential direction. The circumferential fibers resist axial loads which are converted into hoop stresses, whereas the radial fibers resist shear forces [11, 13–15]. Hoop stress, whereupon axial load is dispersed radially, can only be possible with rigid fixation points anteriorly and posteriorly. Thus, it becomes apparent why meniscal horn avulsions that fail to heal essentially render the meniscus impotent. It is important to mention

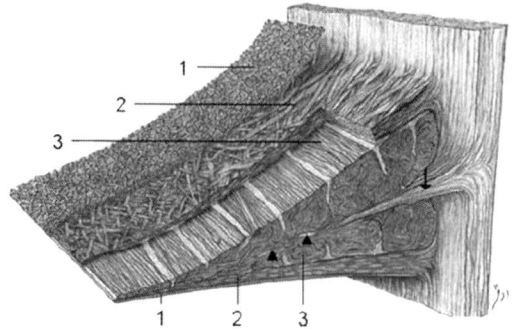

Fig. 1.1 Cross-sectional view of meniscus demonstrating orientations of fibers. (1) Superficial mesh layer, (2) lamellar network, and (3) circumferential fibers. *Arrows* indicate radially oriented fibers. (Reprinted with permission from Springer: Petersen, W. and B. Tillmann, Collagenous fibril texture of the human knee joint menisci. Anat Embryol (Berl), 1998. 197(4): p. 317–24)

that meniscal tears, when repaired, heal with scar and with some shortening of width. The native, delicate, and fine architecture of the meniscus is never fully restored. Therefore, meniscus repair, while certainly less injurious to knee homeostasis than meniscal resection, will never fully afford the same chondroprotection as preservation of native tissue.

The composition of the extracellular matrix of meniscus is generally accepted to be roughly 70 % water and 30 % dry weight in the mature knee [6]. In the young knee, water content is much higher until the composition of the collagen and proteoglycans increases to levels typically seen in adults [16]. The dry weight portion can be divided into collagen, noncollagenous proteins, and proteoglycans. The predominate collagen is type I collagen with varying degrees of type II, II, V, and VI collagens [6]. Elastin is an integral noncollagenous protein that serves to aid in the overall structure and stability of the menisci and comprises 0.6 % of the dry weight [6, 17]. Proteoglycans are formed by a protein core to which one or more glycosaminoglycan (GAG) chains are attached. In comparison to articular cartilage found elsewhere, the proteoglycan content in the meniscus is significantly less among the same species [18, 19]. The predominate GAGs are chondroitin 6-sulfate, chondroitin 4-sulfate, keratin sulfate, and dermatan sulfate [6].

Macroanatomy

Medial Meniscus

The medial meniscus has a C-shape appearance and covers approximately 50 % of the medial tibial plateau. The size of the medial meniscus approximates 4.4 cm in length and 3.1 cm in width. Meniscal dimensions have been strongly correlated to a patient's gender, height, and weight and are important to take into account when considering meniscal transplantation [20]. The posterior horn is larger than the anterior horn in the anteroposterior dimension. The medial meniscus has multiple attachments within the medial compartment. It is attached at the anterior and posterior horns through bony attachments and along the periphery to the joint capsule. The anterior attachment has been shown to have multiple variations with four distinct types currently described [21]. Posteriorly, the attachment is anterior to the attachment of the posterior cruciate ligament. The coronary ligament attaches the inferior aspect of the meniscus to the tibia [22]. Unique to the medial meniscus is its attachment to the deep fibers of the medial collateral ligament.

The medial meniscus can translate approximately 5 mm in the anterior-posterior plane which allows for adequate femoral rollback during knee flexion [23, 24]. Because of the relatively firm attachments to surrounding soft tissue and bony structures, the medial meniscus provides anteroposterior stability to the knee, which is most evident in cases of anterior cruciate ligament (ACL) deficiency. The posterior horn of the medial meniscus acts as a wedge to block anterior translation and thus is an important agonist to the ACL. In the presence of ACL injury, the posterior horn of the medial meniscus experiences large stresses that can lead to attritional tears over time. Such tears can nullify the hoop forces that contribute to the shock dissipation characteristics of the meniscus. In addition, a combined ACL deficiency and medial meniscectomy can lead to an average 58 % increase in anterior tibial translation [25].

Lateral Meniscus

The lateral meniscus has a more circular or ovoid appearance and covers approximately 70 % of the lateral tibial plateau. Dimensions of the lateral meniscus approximate 3.6 cm in length and 2.9 cm in width. Similar to the medial meniscus, variations in sizing is largely correlated with gender, height, and weight. The anterior and posterior attachments of the lateral meniscus are much closer together than that of the medial meniscus (see Fig. 1.2). Anteriorly, the lateral meniscus attaches adjacent to the anterior cruciate ligament. Posteriorly, the attachment is behind the intercondylar eminence anterior to the attachment of the posterior horn of the medial meniscus. In addition to the bony attachments of the anterior and posterior horns are the meniscofemoral ligaments and the popliteomeniscal fasciculi. The ligament of Wrisberg passes posterior to the PCL and attaches to the femur, while the ligament of Humphrey passes anterior to the PCL. In some discoid variants, the bony attachment of the posterior horn is completely absent, and the ligament of Wrisberg becomes the primary posterior stabilizer. The popliteomeniscal fasciculi connect the lateral meniscus to the popliteus tendon and joint capsule, adding to the stability of the lateral meniscus [26]. Overall, the lateral meniscus is more loosely affixed to the lateral compartment than the medial meniscus is within the medial compartment. The lateral meniscus can translate approximately 11 mm during normal knee kinematics [24]. This increased mobility allows the increased tibiofemoral excursion seen in the lateral compartment.

Discoid Meniscus Variants

Variants of the anatomic appearance of the menisci are much more common in the lateral meniscus with a reported incidence between 1.5 and 16.6 %, and of these, 5–20 % occur bilaterally [27–34]. The Watanabe classification is used to describe discoid variants of the lateral meniscus. Three distinct types exist: (a) incomplete, (b) complete, and (c) Wrisberg variant (see Fig. 1.3). Discoid menisci are thicker, often lack

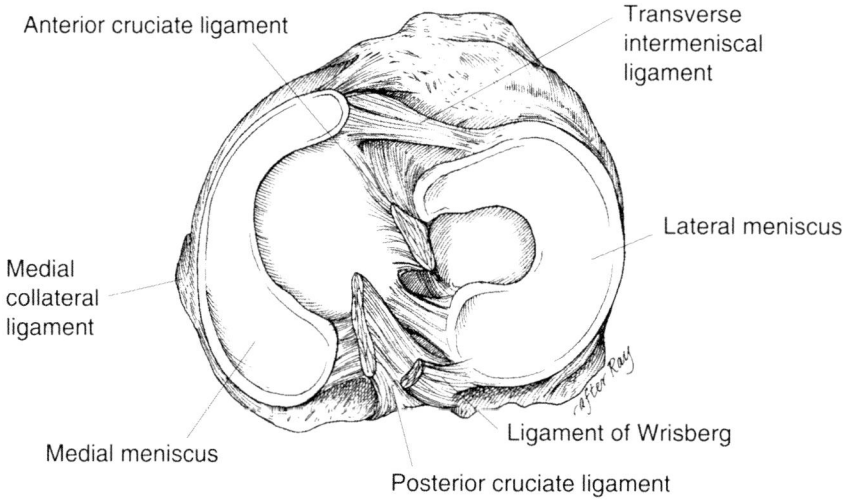

Anterior cruciate ligament

Transverse
intermeniscal
ligament

Lateral meniscus

Medial
collateral
ligament

Medial meniscus

Ligament of Wrisberg

Posterior cruciate ligament

Fig. 1.2 Meniscal Anatomy and relationship to important structures of the knee joint. (Reprinted with permission from: Pagnani MJ, Warren RF, Arnoczky SP, Wickiewicz TL: Anatomy of the knee, in Nicholas JA, Hershman EB, eds: The Lower Extremity and Spine in Sports Medicine, 2nd ed. St. Louis, MO, Mosby, 1995, pp 581–614)

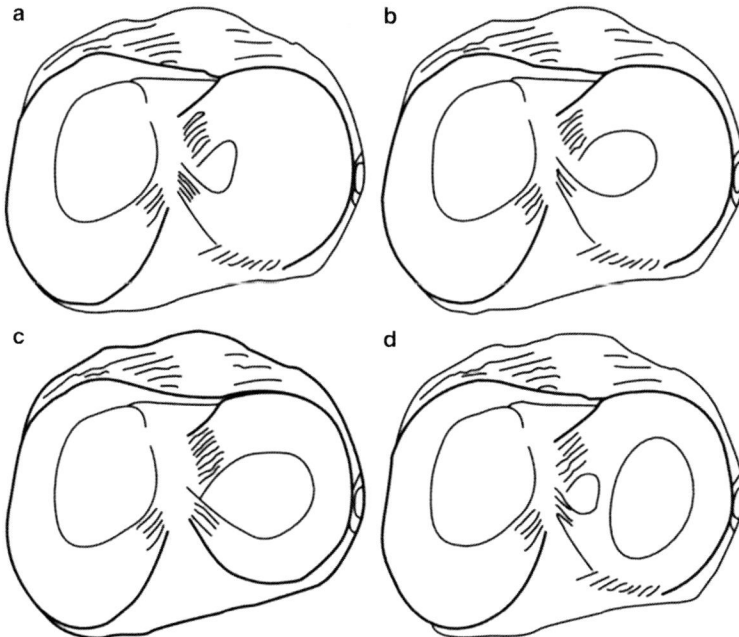

Fig. 1.3 Watanabe's classification of discoid meniscus. (Reprinted with permission from Springer: Atay OA, Yılgör İÇ, Doral MN. Lateral Meniscal Variations and Treatment Strategies. In: Doral MN, editor. Sports Injuries. Heidelberg. Springer-Verlag Berlin Heidelberg; 2012)

a consolidated matrix, lack the normal tapered central contour seen in normal menisci, and, in the case of the Wrisberg variant, lack normal bony attachments, predisposing them to failure. Majority of the time, however, discoid variants are asymptomatic and are incidental findings.

Meniscomeniscal Ligaments

In addition to the tibial, meniscofemoral, and capsular attachments listed previously, there also variable attachments that connect the two menisci together. There are four normal meniscomeniscal attachments that have been described: the anterior and posterior transverse meniscal ligaments and the medial and lateral oblique meniscomeniscal ligaments. The most prevalent by far of these is the anterior transverse meniscal ligament which is present in roughly 58 % of patients. The orientation of the fibers is such that the anterior horn of the medial meniscus is attached to the anterior horn of the lateral meniscus and three variants have been described (see Fig. 1.4) [35]. The overall significance of these attachments is debated, with some investigators ascribing a significant stabilizing role to the anterior horn of the medial meniscus. However, it is important to keep these in mind when evaluating MRI's which can easily be misinterpreted as an anterior horn meniscal tear [36].

Vascular Supply

The main vascular supply to the meniscus comes primarily from the superior and inferior geniculate arteries; the middle geniculate supplies a portion of the anterior and posterior horns. At birth the entire meniscus is highly vascular [5]. This changes rather rapidly with normal development, and by the age of 9 months, the inner one-third becomes avascular. By the age of 10, the vascular supply to the meniscus approximates that of the adult meniscus. The superior and inferior geniculate arteries form a perimeniscal network of capillaries that infiltrate the periphery of the meniscus. This plexus of capillaries supplies 10–30 % of the medial meniscus and 10–25 % of the lateral meniscus [37] (see Fig. 1.5). A small area immediately adjacent to the popliteus is completely avascular [37]. In addition to the vascular supply, a small amount of nutrients are supplied by diffusion of synovial fluid [23].

Clinically, the vasculature is a very important consideration when addressing meniscal tears. The regional variability in vascularity dictates the

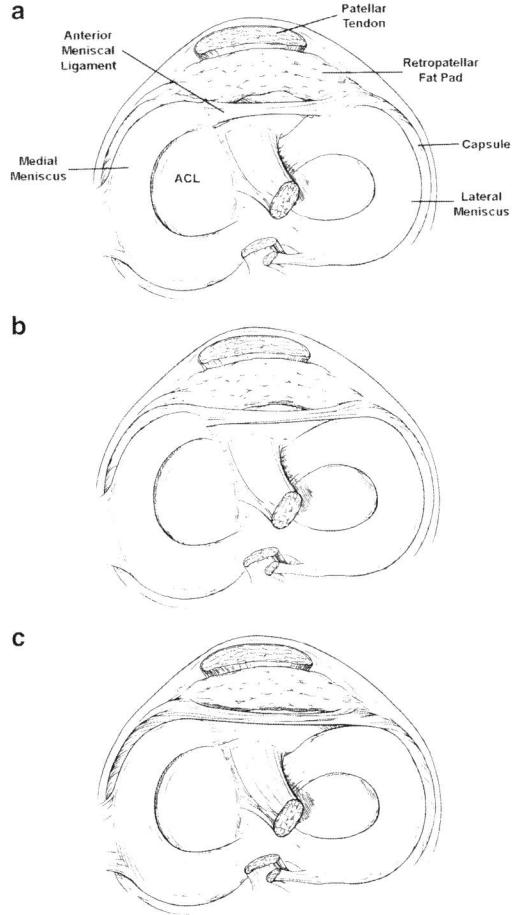

Fig. 1.4 Variations in the attachment of the anterior transverse meniscal ligament. (**a**) Type I attachments to anterior horn of medial meniscus and anterior margin of lateral meniscus. (**b**) Type II attachments to the medial aspect of the anterior horn of the medial meniscus and the joint capsule anterior to the lateral meniscus. (**c**) Type III attachments to the joint capsule anterior to both the medial and lateral meniscus, no direct meniscal attachments. (Reprinted from [35] with permission from SAGE Publications)

healing capability of a tear. The relatively vascular red–red zone of the peripheral meniscus has healing potential and may be amenable to repair (see Fig. 1.4). Conversely, the white–white zone of the inner meniscus is relatively avascular. The healing potential in this area is low, and tears are usually treated with meniscectomy rather than attempted repair. These red–red and white–white regions are separated by a transitional red–white zone which has intermediate healing potential

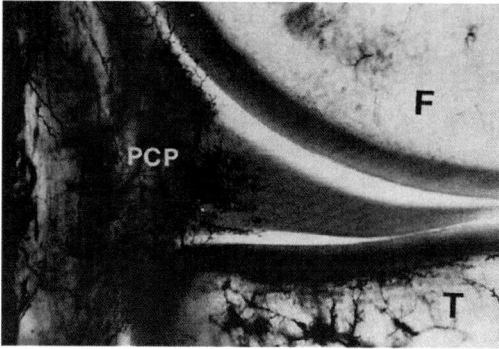

Fig. 1.5 India ink demonstrating vasculature of the meniscus. (Reprinted from [37] with permission from SAGE Publications)

Neuroanatomy

The neuroanatomy of the meniscus is similar to the vascular anatomy in that neural elements are contained within the periphery only, leaving the central portion devoid of any neural elements. In awake patients, probing the central area of the meniscus produces no pain, whereas probing the peripheral portions can elicit pain and discomfort [38]. To understand how this correlates clinically, the analogy of getting a haircut can be used. When the hair is cut there is no pain; however, if you were to tug on the hair, pain is usually felt. Thus inner rim tears can clearly evoke discomfort. In addition to sensory fibers, mechanoreceptors are also found in the peripheral portion of the meniscus. Mechanoreceptors are important in proprioception in the knee joint [23], continually relaying to the brain input regarding knee position. The loss of proprioception with loss of meniscal tissue is perhaps an additional reason why meniscectomy may lead to osteoarthritis.

Summary and Conclusions

The menisci are fibrocartilaginous structures within the knee joint that play important roles in the normal function of the knee. The menisci arise from mesenchymal progenitor cells in the limb bud and become distinct structures by the 8th week of gestation. The fibrochondrocyte is the primary cell type of the meniscus, and these cells are arranged in a complex manner which, along with the extracellular matrix, forms the basis of the mechanical properties of the meniscus. The extracellular matrix is composed of ~ 70 % water and ~30 % collagen and proteoglycans. The medial and lateral menisci differ in size and shape, and their dimension is correlated to gender, height, and weight. The menisci are attached within the joint primarily by bony attachments of the anterior and posterior horns with accessory structures providing some stability. The medial meniscus has more soft tissue and bony connections than does the lateral meniscus and, therefore, plays a more important role in joint stability, especially in the case of ACL insufficiency. While the entire meniscus is vascular early in development, the vascular supply in the adult meniscus occurs only in the periphery which has important implications in the treatment of meniscal tears. The majority of the meniscus is void of any neural elements; however, mechanoreceptors and sensory fibers can be found in the periphery and contribute to proprioception of the knee and along with nociception—the recognition of pain seen in meniscal tears.

References

1. Gardner E, O'Rahilly R. The early development of the knee joint in staged human embryos. J Anat. 1968;102(Pt 2):289–99.
2. Hyde G, Boot-Handford RP, Wallis GA. Col2a1 lineage tracing reveals that the meniscus of the knee joint has a complex cellular origin. J Anat. 2008;213(5):531–8.
3. Gray DJ, Gardner E. Prenatal development of the human knee and superior tibiofibular joints. Am J Anat. 1950;86(2):235–87.
4. O'Rahilly R. The early prenatal development of the human knee joint. J Anat. 1951;85(2):166–70.
5. Clark CR, Ogden JA. Development of the menisci of the human knee joint. Morphological changes and their potential role in childhood meniscal injury. J Bone Joint Surg Am. 1983;65(4):538–47.
6. McDevitt CA, Webber RJ. The ultrastructure and biochemistry of meniscal cartilage. Clin Orthop Relat Res. 1990;252:8–18.

7. Cheung HS. Distribution of type I, II, III and V in the pepsin solubilized collagens in bovine menisci. Connect Tissue Res. 1987;16(4):343–56.
8. Messner K, Gao J. The menisci of the knee joint. Anatomical and functional characteristics, and a rationale for clinical treatment. J Anat. 1998;193(Pt 2): 161–78.
9. Hellio Le Graverand MP, et al. The cells of the rabbit meniscus: their arrangement, interrelationship, morphological variations and cytoarchitecture. J Anat. 2001;198(Pt 5):525–35.
10. Ghadially FN, et al. Ultrastructure of rabbit semilunar cartilages. J Anat. 1978;125(Pt 3):499–517.
11. Petersen W, Tillmann B. Collagenous fibril texture of the human knee joint menisci. Anat Embryol (Berl). 1998;197(4):317–24.
12. Wagner HJ. Architecture of collagen fibers in the meniscus of the human knee joint, with special reference to the medial meniscus and its connection to the articular ligaments. Z Mikrosk Anat Forsch. 1976; 90(2):302–24.
13. Beaupre A, et al. Knee menisci. Correlation between microstructure and biomechanics. Clin Orthop Relat Res. 1986;208:72–5.
14. Bullough PG, et al. The strength of the menisci of the knee as it relates to their fine structure. J Bone Joint Surg Br. 1970;52(3):564–7.
15. Shrive NG, O'Connor JJ, Goodfellow JW. Load-bearing in the knee joint. Clin Orthop Relat Res. 1978;131:279–87.
16. Ghosh P, Taylor TK. The knee joint meniscus. A fibrocartilage of some distinction. Clin Orthop Relat Res. 1987;224:52–63.
17. Pierschbacher MD, Hayman EG, Ruoslahti E. The cell attachment determinant in fibronectin. J Cell Biochem. 1985;28(2):115–26.
18. Adams ME, Muir H. The glycosaminoglycans of canine menisci. Biochem J. 1981;197(2):385–9.
19. Atencia LJ, et al. Cartilage content of an immature dog. Connect Tissue Res. 1989;18(4):235–42.
20. Van Thiel GS, et al. Meniscal allograft size can be predicted by height, weight, and gender. Arthroscopy. 2009;25(7):722–7.
21. Berlet GC, Fowler PJ. The anterior horn of the medial meniscus. An anatomic study of its insertion. Am J Sports Med. 1998;26(4):540–3.
22. Johnson DL, et al. Insertion-site anatomy of the human menisci: gross, arthroscopic, and topographical anatomy as a basis for meniscal transplantation. Arthroscopy. 1995;11(4):386–94.
23. Greis PE, et al. Meniscal injury: I. Basic science and evaluation. J Am Acad Orthop Surg. 2002;10(3): 168–76.
24. Thompson WO, et al. Tibial meniscal dynamics using three-dimensional reconstruction of magnetic resonance images. Am J Sports Med. 1991;19(3):210–5. discussion 215-6.
25. Levy IM, et al. The effect of lateral meniscectomy on motion of the knee. J Bone Joint Surg Am. 1989; 71(3):401–6.
26. Simonian PT, et al. Popliteomeniscal fasciculi and lateral meniscal stability. Am J Sports Med. 1997; 25(6):849–53.
27. Rao SK, Sripathi RP. Clinical, radiologic and arthroscopic assessment and treatment of bilateral discoid lateral meniscus. Knee Surg Sports Traumatol Arthrosc. 2007;15(5):597–601.
28. Aichroth PM, Patel DV, Marx CL. Congenital discoid lateral meniscus in children. A follow-up study and evolution of management. J Bone Joint Surg Br. 1991;73(6):932–6.
29. Bellier G, et al. Lateral discoid menisci in children. Arthroscopy. 1989;5(1):52–6.
30. Pellacci F, et al. Lateral discoid meniscus: treatment and results. Arthroscopy. 1992;8(4):526–30.
31. Ikeuchi H. Arthroscopic treatment of the discoid lateral meniscus. Technique and long-term results. Clin Orthop Relat Res. 1982;167:19–28.
32. Dickhaut SC, DeLee JC. The discoid lateral-meniscus syndrome. J Bone Joint Surg Am. 1982;64(7):1068–73.
33. Wojtys EM, Chan DB. Meniscus structure and function. Instr Course Lect. 2005;54:323–30.
34. Kocher MS, Klingele K, Rassman SO. Meniscal disorders: normal, discoid, and cysts. Orthop Clin North Am. 2003;34(3):329–40.
35. Nelson EW, LaPrade RF. The anterior intermeniscal ligament of the knee. An anatomic study. Am J Sports Med. 2000;28(1):74–6.
36. Zivanovic S. Menisco-meniscal ligaments of the human knee joint. Anat Anz. 1974;135(1–2):35–42.
37. Arnoczky SP, Warren RF. Microvasculature of the human meniscus. Am J Sports Med. 1982;10(2):90–5.
38. Dye SF, Vaupel GL, Dye CC. Conscious neurosensory mapping of the internal structures of the human knee without intraarticular anesthesia. Am J Sports Med. 1998;26(6):773–7.

Physical Examination for Meniscus Tears

Kevin J. McHale, Min Jung Park,
and Fotios Paul Tjoumakaris

Abbreviations

ACL	Anterior cruciate ligament
ER	External rotation
IR	Internal rotation
PCL	Posterior cruciate ligament
LCL	Lateral collateral ligament
MCL	Medial collateral ligament
PLC	Posterolateral corner

Introduction

Meniscus injuries, both from athletic activities and activities of daily living, are a common reason of referral for orthopedic evaluation. With an annual incidence of approximately 61 per 100,000 individuals in the general population, meniscus tears are one of the most common injuries to the knee and should often be included at the top of the differential diagnosis for patients presenting with knee pain [1]. While imaging techniques are playing an increasingly important role in confirming the diagnosis of meniscus injury, physicians must be capable of performing a thorough history and physical examination as it relates to the meniscus to determine when obtaining advanced imaging will be advantageous. This chapter will provide a review of the basic approach to the physical examination of the knee with a particular focus on the evaluation for meniscus tears.

History

Prior to performing the physical examination, it is essential that the physician obtain a focused history to facilitate the identification of a meniscus tear. The history is critical to determining optimal treatment for patients and determining the type of meniscus tear (acute versus chronic/degenerative). In the words of esteemed physician, Sir William Osler, "Listen to your patient, he is telling you the diagnosis," patients with sudden onset of pain in the setting of a twisting injury to the knee are more likely to require further diagnostic testing and, perhaps, surgical intervention. Patients with an insidious onset of pain without preceding injury may have underlying articular cartilage degeneration and joint wear that will more than likely dictate the treatment strategy. Several valuable features of the history include location and character of pain (medial versus lateral joint line), mechanism of injury, ability to bear weight, locking or instability sensations, appreciation of a "pop" at the time of injury, and

K.J. McHale, M.D. (✉) • M.J. Park, M.D., M.M.Sc.
Department of Orthopaedic Surgery, Hospital of the
University of Pennsylvania, 3400 Spruce Street,
Silverstein 2, Philadelphia, PA 19104, USA
e-mail: Kevin.mchale@uphs.upenn.edu

F.P. Tjoumakaris, M.D.
Department of Orthopaedic Surgery, Jefferson
Medical College, Rothman Institute Orthopaedics,
Egg Harbor Township, NJ, USA

history of previous knee injury. Patients may report pain with directional change during walking, difficulty squatting, as well as pain with ascending or descending stairs. Patients with medial meniscal tears may relate a history of pain when crossing their legs. Similarly, sudden pain localized to the joint-line when catching one's foot on an irregular surface is also indicative of meniscal pathology. While meniscus tears are often associated with mechanical symptoms such as "clicking" or "catching," these symptoms may also be caused by intra-articular loose bodies from chondral injuries or from abnormal patellofemoral mechanics. Patella maltracking is commonly referred to as "pseudolocking" because sudden patella displacement can indeed mimic meniscal symptoms subjectively. A complaint of "locking" with a mechanical block to extension may be associated with a displaced bucket-handle meniscus tear. Degenerative meniscus tears tend to occur in the absence of antecedent trauma in patients older than 40 years of age and are often associated with a history of joint-line pain and swelling with or without mechanical symptoms.

The clinical history also assists with the development of a comprehensive differential diagnosis that includes alternative or additional causes of knee pain. For example, anterior cruciate ligament (ACL) tears are often a result of a noncontact pivoting injury associated with an audible "pop" and immediate onset of pain and swelling. Posterior cruciate ligament (PCL) injuries can be caused by a direct blow to the proximal tibia, such as from a dashboard during a motor vehicle collision. A mechanism of injury that includes a varus or valgus stress to the knee with a resultant sensation of instability may be associated with lateral collateral ligament (LCL) or medial collateral ligament (MCL) injuries, respectively.

When evaluating patients with knee pain, physicians should keep a high clinical suspicion for meniscus injury even after an alternative source of pain has been identified. Meniscus tears often occur in combination with other knee injuries. Approximately one-third of all meniscus tears are associated with ACL injuries [1]. In the setting of an acute ACL tear, lateral meniscus tears

occur more frequently than medial meniscus tears. In contrast, medial meniscus injuries are more common in knees with a chronic ACL deficiency due to the role of the posterior horn of the medial meniscus as a secondary restraint to anteroposterior translation. Injuries to the menisci are also common in the setting of multiligament knee injuries as well as tibial plateau and femoral shaft fractures [2]. Treatment of meniscus injuries in this setting is dependent upon the treatment of the ligament disruption or fracture and is typically delayed until the primary issues are addressed.

General Examination

The physical examination always begins with an assessment of height and weight. The patient's body mass index should be calculated as load bearing across the knee joint is affected by body weight and characteristic tears occur in larger framed individuals. For example, degenerative meniscal tears occur in the setting of obesity. Furthermore, women with a high body mass index have a proclivity for meniscal root avulsion. Patients should be offered examination shorts so that assessment of both knees can be performed. These garments should be comfortable and rest above the knee for easy inspection during the examination.

Inspection of the knee begins with evaluation of gait. The knee should smoothly transition through a sequence of motions during the normal gait cycle. During swing phase, the quadriceps contracts to extend the knee and to begin accelerating the lower limb from a flexed position. At midpoint of swing phase, the hamstrings begin to contract to decelerate the lower limb in preparation for heel strike. The knee reaches full extension at heel strike and then remains flexed through the foot flat and midstance portion of the stance phase. Push off then marks the end of stance phase and the start of the next swing phase [3]. Patients with meniscus tears or degenerative changes in the knee often experience pain during the stance phase of gait. Push off can be particularly troublesome for patients with advanced chondrosis, since the gait phase is where tibiofemoral joint reactive forces peak [4]. These patients tend to ambulate with an antalgic gait, shortening the amount of time spent on the affected extremity during stance phase. Patients with an associated ligamentous injury may also widen their gait to accommodate knee instability [3]. The physician should next evaluate the alignment of the knee joint. The normal knee has a slight valgus alignment with a tibiofemoral angle of approximately 6°. Varus or valgus malalignment of the knee should be noted as it alters normal knee kinematics by shifting the load bearing axis medially or laterally, respectively. Varus malalignment increases stress applied to the medial meniscus while valgus malalignment heightens contact pressure across the lateral meniscus. As a result, medial and lateral meniscus tears have been correlated with varus and valgus malalignment, respectively [5]. Furthermore, alignment promotes meniscal "dependency": that is, a varus knee will have more inherent dependence on the medial meniscus to dissipate load.

When examining the alignment of the knee, the clinician should also assess the quadriceps (Q) angle. The Q angle is the angle between the axis of the extensor mechanism (anterosuperior iliac spine to the mid-patella) and the axis of the patellar tendon (mid-patella to the tibial tubercle) with the knee in extension. The average Q angle is 10° in men and 15° in women. Abnormalities in the Q angle may result in patellar maltracking [6]. Similarly, a "J" sign should be noted, whereupon a quadriceps contraction leads to lateral excursion of the patella in extension. This indicates maltracking due to an excessive Q angle and/or trochlear dysplasia.

Inspection of the knee joint should also include assessment of the skin and muscle tone. Skin abnormalities such as abrasions, lacerations, ecchymosis, and erythema can provide important information regarding the etiology of knee pain. Asymmetry of muscle contours above the knee, particularly atrophy of the quadriceps, may indicate disuse after injury and can help the clinician to determine chronicity.

Palpation of the Knee Joint

The physician should thoroughly palpate the bony and soft tissue structures of the affected and unaffected knees, paying particular attention to areas of focal tenderness and swelling. Palpation of the knee is best performed with the patient lying supine on the examination table to allow for full unrestricted range of motion. The clinician can begin with palpation of the anterior structures of the knee including the quadriceps tendon, patella, and infrapatellar tendon. Any focal tenderness or palpable defects noted during the examination could indicate an injury to the extensor mechanism. When evaluating the anterior structures, the clinician should also note any warmth, erythema, or tenderness overlying the regions of the suprapatellar, prepatellar, or infrapatellar bursas, as they can be significant sources of pain when inflamed secondary to infection or overuse.

After assessment of the anterior knee structures, the physician can address the medial aspect of the knee joint. Careful attention should be paid to the palpation of the medial meniscus at the upper edge of the medial tibial plateau (Fig. 2.1a) and the MCL extending from the medial femoral epicondyle to the medial proximal tibia. Tenderness to palpation along the posterior medial joint line can indicate a medial meniscus tear, MCL injury, or medial compartment osteoarthritis. On the posteromedial aspect of the knee, the sartorius, gracilis, and semitendinosus tendons can be palpated as they cross the knee joint prior to inserting on the anteromedial proximal tibia at the pes anserine bursa, which may become inflamed and cause pain with knee motion [3]. Palpation of the anteromedial joint line relative to the distal femur can also indicate any subtle posterior subluxation of the tibia. Normal tibiofemoral step-off is approximately 10 mm with the tibia being anterior to the femur with the knee at 90° of flexion. Decreased step-off can indicate injury to the posterior cruciate ligament and posterior capsular structures [7]. Anteromedial tenderness may also be present when patella

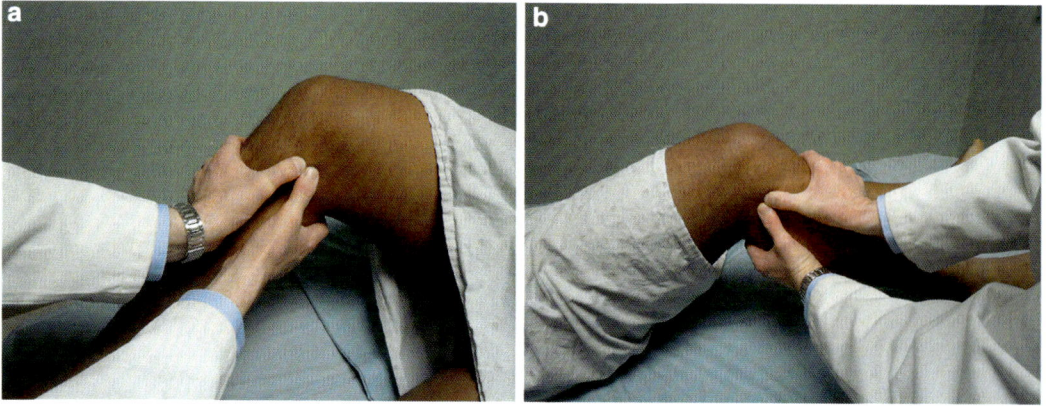

Fig. 2.1 Palpation of the meniscus. (a) Palpation of medial meniscus. (b) Palpation of lateral meniscus

maltracking is present and may represent fat pad irritation, synovitis, or tension on medial patellofemoral ligaments.

The lateral knee must also be evaluated carefully with palpation. Analogous to the medial aspect of the knee, the lateral meniscus can be palpated at the upper edge of the lateral tibial plateau (Fig. 2.1b) and the LCL can be palpated as it extends from the lateral femoral epicondyle to the fibular head. Tenderness to palpation along the lateral joint line can indicate a lateral meniscus tear, LCL injury, or lateral compartment osteoarthritis. The biceps femoris and iliotibial tract can also be palpated as they cross the knee joint to insert on the fibular head and lateral tibial tubercle, respectively. Palpation of the lateral joint line can be facilitated by placing the knee in a crossed position, or the "figure of four" position. This places a varus moment on the knee, opening up the lateral compartment. The LCL can easily be palpated running from the lateral epicondyle to the fibular head, and posterior to this structure on the joint line is the lateral meniscus body and posterior horn segment. Care must be taken to differentiate joint-line tenderness from popliteus tendonitis (more proximal) or iliotibial friction band syndrome (more proximal).

The final step in the palpation of the knee joint is the assessment for intra-articular effusions. While the absence of indentations adjacent to the infrapatellar tendon implies the presence of a large intra-articular effusion, specific physical examination maneuvers can assist with the detection of more subtle effusions. The first maneuver involves the creation of a fluid wave to detect an effusion. With the knee extended, intra-articular fluid can be milked into the suprapatellar pouch by sliding the hand proximally along the medial aspect of the patella. Next, this fluid can be compressed out of the suprapatellar pouch by sliding the hand distally along the lateral aspect of the patella. A fluid bulge can be seen medial to the patella with this lateral compression in the presence of an intra-articular effusion. Another maneuver to detect an effusion involves the ballottement of the patella in the presence of an effusion. One hand is used to compress fluid from the suprapatellar pouch to beneath the patella while the second hand squeezes fluid from the inferior aspect of the joint to beneath the patella. A finger can then be used to depress the patella, which will feel as if it is bouncing on the underlying effusion [8].

Range of Motion

The physician should evaluate both active and passive range of motion of the knee joint. Normal knee extension ranges from 0° to -10°, and normal knee flexion ranges from 130° to 150°. The patella should be observed for appropriate tracking with active and passive knee range of motion. Patellofemoral crepitus can often be observed with range of motion in the presence of patellofemoral osteoarthritis. Crepitus and/or pain in early flexion indicates more distal patella disease. Joint pain that is present during both active and passive range of motion is often associated with intra-articular pathology while pain that is present only with active range of motion has a higher likelihood of being related to an extra-articular soft tissue disorder [8].

Joint Stability

The assessment of joint stability is an essential part of every orthopedic knee examination. When evaluating joint stability, the physician should perform a series of maneuvers to both the affected and unaffected knee to test the collateral and cruciate ligaments for laxity. The MCL is best evaluated with the patient supine by applying a valgus stress to the knee joint both with the knee in 30° of flexion and in full extension. The LCL can be assessed in a similar manner by applying a varus stress to the knee joint in 30° of flexion and full extension. By stressing the knee in flexion and extension, the clinician can test the collateral ligaments both in isolation and in combination with the secondary stabilizers of the knee. Laxity to valgus or varus stress with the knee in 30° of flexion indicates an isolated injury to the MCL or LCL, respectively. When laxity is also noted to varus or valgus stress with the knee in full extension, one or both cruciate ligaments are likely injured in addition to a collateral ligament [9]. The physical examination maneuvers utilized for the evaluation of the collateral ligaments are summarized in Table 2.1.

The examiner should also consider meniscal pathology when evaluating the stability of the collateral ligaments. When performing isolated varus or valgus stress, pain on the side of compression suggests meniscal injury while pain on the side of distraction implicates ligamentous pathology. As a result, medial knee pain with varus stress and lateral knee pain with valgus stress are concerning for medial and lateral meniscus tears, respectively [10].

The posteromedial and posterolateral complexes of the knee are also important collateral stabilizers of the knee joint. The posterior oblique

Table 2.1 Physical examination of the collateral ligaments

Physical exam test	Technique	Significance
Valgus stress	Valgus stress applied to knee in 30° flexion and full extension	Laxity in 30° flexion indicates isolated MCL injury. Laxity in full extension indicates MCL injury with associated cruciate ligament injury
Varus stress	Varus stress applied to knee in 30° flexion and full extension	Laxity in 30° flexion indicates isolated LCL injury. Laxity in full extension indicates LCL injury with associated cruciate ligament injury

ligament and posteromedial joint capsule of the posteromedial complex prevent excessive antero-medial rotation, while the posterolateral complex (popliteus, fibular collateral ligament, popliteo-fibular ligament, fabellofibular ligament, arcuate complex, and lateral head of the gastrocnemius) prevents excessive posterolateral rotation. The anterior rotation drawer test and dial test are important maneuvers to determine whether pathology in these structures may exist.

The anterior rotation drawer test can be used to assess for both posteromedial and posterolateral instability. This maneuver is performed by applying an anterior drawer force to the tibia with the knee flexed at 90°. The anterior force is first applied in the neutral position, then with 15° of tibial internal rotation, and finally with 30° of tibial external rotation. Increased subluxation of the tibial plateau in reference to the femoral condyles in neutral position that is accentuated by external rotation and decreased by internal rotation is indicative of anteromedial instability. Anterior tibial subluxation in neutral position that is increased with internal rotation and decreased by external rotation is indicative of posterolateral instability [11].

The dial test can also be used to assess for posterolateral instability. This maneuver can be performed both with the patient supine and prone. With either position, the examiner should use one hand to grasp each of the patient's feet and externally rotate the lower legs simultaneously first at 30° of knee flexion and then at 90° of knee flexion.

Table 2.2 Physical examination of the anterior cruciate ligament

Physical exam test	Technique	Significance	Reliability
Lachman test	Anterior proximal tibial translation with knee in 30° flexion	Soft end point or increased translation compared to contralateral knee is concerning for ACL injury	Sensitivity: 80–99 % [12–17] Specificity: 95 % [14]
Anterior drawer	Anterior proximal tibial translation with knee in 90° flexion	Soft end point or increased translation compared to contralateral knee is concerning for ACL injury	Sensitivity: 22.2–95.24 % [12–14, 16, 17] Specificity: >97 % [14]
Pivot shift	Knee passively flexed with lower extremity in slight internal rotation (IR) while valgus stress applied	An appreciable "clunk" at 30° knee flexion from spontaneous reduction of displaced tibial plateau is suggestive of ACL injury	Sensitivity: 35–98.4 % [13, 14] Specificity: >98 % [13, 14]

A positive dial test is indicated by asymmetric external rotation (>15°) of the symptomatic extremity when compared to the asymptomatic extremity. A positive dial test performed at 30° of knee flexion is concerning for an isolated PLC injury. A positive dial test both at 30 and 90° of knee flexion is concerning for a PCL injury in addition to a PLC injury [6]. The prone position may be more favorable since it safeguards against excessive anteromedial tibial subluxation.

After the collateral ligaments are evaluated, attention should then be turned to examination of the cruciate ligaments. The physical examination tests used during the evaluation for ACL injury, including the Lachman test, anterior drawer, and pivot shift test, are summarized in Table 2.2. The Lachman test is the most sensitive and specific physical examination maneuver for the detection of an ACL injury with reported sensitivity ranging from 80 % to 99 % [12–17] and a specificity of 95 % [14]. This test is performed with the patient placed in the supine position with the knee flexed at approximately 20–30°. With one hand stabilizing the femur, the examiner's second hand is used to briskly anteriorly translate the proximal tibia with respect to the femur. A soft end point to anterior translation or greater translation when compared to the unaffected knee is considered a positive Lachman test and is concerning for a possible ACL injury [17].

The anterior drawer test may also be used to assist with the identification of an ACL injury. In this test, the patient is positioned supine with the hip flexed at 45° and the knee flexed at 90°.

The examiner places both hands on the proximal tibia with thumbs on the anterior tibial plateau and remaining fingers wrapped posteriorly. The lower extremity can be stabilized by sitting on the patient's foot. An anterior translational force is then applied to the proximal tibia in relation to the femur. Analogous to the Lachman test, the anterior drawer test is positive for injury to the ACL injury when it results in a soft end point or increased anterior translation of the proximal tibia when compared to the unaffected side [9]. Reported sensitivity of this test is much more variable, ranging from 22.2 % to 95.24 % [12–17]. The specificity of the anterior drawer has been reported as greater than 97 % [14].

The pivot shift test is another effective maneuver for the detection of an ACL tear. This test is based on the anterior subluxation of the lateral tibial plateau relative to the femoral condyle that occurs with full knee extension in the presence of an ACL injury. A positive pivot shift test detects the spontaneous reduction of the tibial plateau with flexion of an ACL deficient knee. To perform the pivot shift test, the examiner uses one hand on the patient's ankle to raise the lower extremity with the knee in full extension and slight internal rotation. The examiner then applies a valgus stress to the knee joint while passively flexing the knee. A positive test will result in a profound clunk at approximately 30° of flexion when the displaced tibial plateau spontaneously reduces beneath the femoral condyle [18]. The sensitivity of the pivot shift test has also been reported to have variable results (35 % to 98.4 %) [13, 14]. The specificity

Table 2.3 Physical examination of the posterior cruciate ligament

Posterior sag sign	Inspection of bilateral proximal tibias with 90° knee flexion and patient supine	Loss of 1 cm anterior step-off of medial proximal tibial plateau in relation to femoral condyle is concerning for PCL injury	Sensitivity: 79 % [19] Specificity: 100 % [19]
Posterior drawer	Posterior proximal tibial translation with knee in 90° flexion	Soft end point or increased translation compared to contralateral knee is concerning for PCL injury	Sensitivity: 51–100 % [5, 18, 19] Specificity: 99 % [19]
Quadriceps active test	Attempted active knee extension from 90° flexion against resistance	Anterior shift of proximal tibial plateau >2 mm suggestive of PCL injury	Sensitivity: 54–98 % [19, 20] Specificity: 97–100 % [19, 20]
Dial test	Simultaneous external rotation (ER) of bilateral lower legs with 30° and 90° knee flexion	Asymmetric ER (>15°) at 30° is suggestive of an isolated PLC injury. Asymmetric ER at 30° and 90° is suggestive of a PCL injury in addition to a PLC injury	

of this test has been reported as 98 % or greater [13, 14].

The PCL can also be evaluated by a variety of clinical examination maneuvers, which are summarized in Table 2.3. The knee should first be inspected for a posterior sag sign, which is indicative of a PCL tear. To test for this sign, the patient is positioned supine with 45° of hip flexion and 90° of knee flexion. In this position, the medial tibial plateau should sit approximately 1 cm anterior to the medial femoral condyle in a knee with an intact PCL. In the presence of a torn PCL, the tibial plateau will sag posteriorly resulting in a loss of this visible step-off and a positive posterior sag sign [7]. The posterior sag sign has been reported to have a sensitivity of 79 % and specificity of 100 % [19].

While maintaining 45° of hip flexion and 90° of knee flexion, a posterior drawer test can then be performed by applying a posterior translational force to the proximal tibia in relation to the femur. The examiner should apply this force using both hands on the proximal tibia with thumbs on the anterior tibial plateau and remaining fingers wrapped posteriorly. The lower extremity can be stabilized during this maneuver by sitting on the patient's foot. A positive posterior drawer test results in increased posterior tibial translation when compared to the unaffected knee and is concerning for PCL injury [9]. The reported sensitivity of the posterior drawer has ranged from

51 % to 100 % [5, 18, 19] while its specificity has been reported as 99 % [19].

The quadriceps active test may also help confirm the posterior tibial displacement of a PCL deficient knee. The patient is maintained in the supine position with 45° of hip flexion and 90° of knee flexion. The foot is again stabilized by the examiner. The patient is then asked to extend the knee against the examiner's resistance. In the presence of a torn PCL, the contraction of the quadriceps muscle results in greater than 2 mm of an anterior shift of the tibial plateau [20]. The quadriceps active test has been shown to have a range of sensitivities from 54 % to 98 % and specificities from 97 % to 100 % [19, 20].

It is essential to look for a posterior sag sign prior to performing cruciate ligament testing to ensure that the tests begin with the normal relationship between the tibial plateau and femoral condyles. An undetected posterior sag of the tibial plateau can lead to a falsely negative posterior drawer test secondary to the lack of additional posterior translation of an already posteriorly subluxed tibia. Additionally, the examiner may falsely diagnose an ACL injury based on an inaccurate Lachman test that resulted in excessive anterior translation due to the initial posterior displacement of the tibial plateau. For this reason, the examiner must be aware of the starting location of the tibial plateau prior to performing cruciate ligament testing.

Evaluation of the Meniscus

After completion of the exam for joint stability, the physician can evaluate the knee for evidence of meniscus injury. As previously described, the examiner can begin by evaluating for medial or lateral joint-line tenderness to palpation. Although joint-line tenderness may result from alternative knee pathology, focal tenderness over the medial or lateral menisci is often present in those with meniscus tears. Joint-line tenderness has been reported to have a sensitivity for detecting meniscal pathology ranging from 55 % to 85 % and a specificity ranging from 29.4 % to 67 % [21–23].

In addition to joint-line tenderness, several provocative maneuvers, summarized in Table 2.4,

can be performed to aid in the diagnosis of meniscus injury. The McMurray test is one of the most widely utilized clinical exam maneuvers to evaluate for meniscus tears. This test is performed with the patient supine (Fig. 2.2). The examiner first brings the knee into full flexion while grasping the patient's foot with one hand and stabilizing the knee with a second hand. The knee is then brought from full flexion to 90° of flexion first with full internal rotation of the tibia and then with full external tibial rotation. A positive test produces an appreciable click in association with a torn meniscus that reproduces the patient's previous painful sensations. Pain or clicking with internal rotation suggests the presence of a lateral meniscus injury while a positive test with external rotation is indicative of medial meniscus injury [26]. This maneuver has been shown to

Table 2.4 Physical examination tests for the detection of meniscus injury

Physical exam test	Technique	Significance	Reliability
Joint-line tenderness	Direct palpation over medial and lateral joint line	Tenderness can indicate a meniscus tear, collateral ligament injury, or DJD	Sensitivity: 55–85 % [21–23] Specificity: 29.4–67 % [21–23]
McMurray test	Range knee from full flexion to 90° of flexion first with full tibial IR and then with full tibial ER	Positive test produces "click" in association with torn meniscus and reproduces patient's painful sensation	Sensitivity: 16–58 % [21–24] Specificity: 77–98 % [22–24]
Apley grind test	Strong ER force applied to knee flexed at 90° at rest, with distraction, and with compression	Joint-line pain with distraction is concerning for ligamentous injury. Joint-line pain with compression is concerning for meniscal pathology	Sensitivity: 13–16 % Specificity: 80–90 % [22, 23]
Bounce home test	Passive full knee extension from flexed position	Loss of terminal extension indicates mechanical block, such as a meniscus tear	
Finochietto test (jump sign)	Anterior proximal tibial translation with knee in 130°–140° flexion	Positive test produces "jump" of torn posterior horn of meniscus with anterior displacement	
Boehler test	Varus and valgus stress applied to knee in almost complete extension	Pain on side of compression is suggestive of meniscus injury	
Thessaly test	Patient internally and externally rotates his or her knee and body while keeping one foot planted with the knee flexed at 5° and then 20°	Joint-line pain with maneuver indicates possible meniscus tear	20° Thessaly test Sensitivity: 89–92 % [25] Specificity: 96–97 % [25]
Childress test	Patient "duck walks" by moving forward with maximal knee flexion	Joint-line pain with maneuver indicates possible meniscus tear	

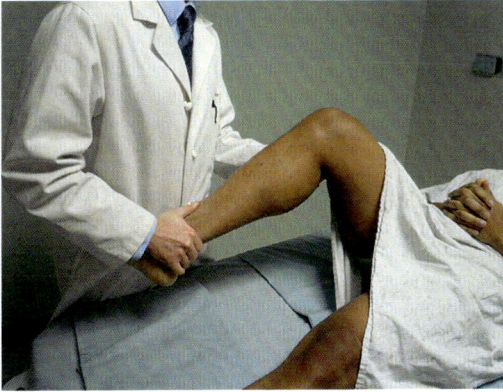

Fig. 2.2 Positioning for McMurray test

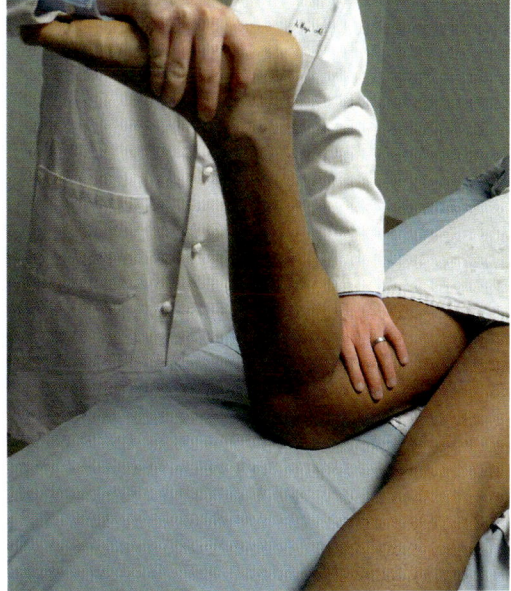

Fig. 2.3 Positioning for Apley grind test

have a modest sensitivity for the detection of meniscus tears with reported values ranging from 16 to 58 % [21–24]. However, the McMurray test is highly specific for meniscus tears, particularly tears of the posterior horn, with specificity values ranging from 77 to 98 % [22–24]. Consequently, this provocative test has continued utility in combination with other physical examination maneuvers for the diagnosis of meniscus injury [26].

The Apley grind test involves a series of provocative maneuvers that also may be used to diagnose a meniscus injury. For this test, the patient is positioned prone (Fig. 2.3). The injured knee is flexed to 90° and a powerful external rotation force is applied to the tibia. This maneuver determines if external rotation of the knee elicits pain. With the thigh stabilized against the examining table, a distraction force is then applied to the lower leg with the knee flexed at a right angle and an external rotation force is again applied. During this test, the physician should note if pain is elicited with distraction and external rotation and if this pain is greater than without distraction. Increased pain with this maneuver indicates a positive distraction test and is concerning for a ligamentous sprain. Pain with distraction also decreases the likelihood that the meniscus is the etiology of knee pain since distraction decreases the compressive force on the meniscus. The examiner next applies a compression force to the knee while applying an external rotation force in 90° of knee flexion. Increased pain with this maneuver indicates a positive compression test

and is concerning for a medial meniscus injury. This series of provocative maneuvers can then be repeated with internal rotation to examine the lateral meniscus [27]. Similar to the McMurray test, the Apley grind test also has been shown to have a relatively low sensitivity (13–16 %) and high specificity (80–90 %) [22, 23].

The bounce home test assesses passive knee range of motion to aid in the diagnosis of meniscus tears. This test begins with the patient positioned supine with full knee flexion. The examiner cups the foot of the affected extremity and allows the knee to passively fall into full extension. When performing this maneuver, the knee should "bounce home" into full extension with a sharp end point. A loss of terminal extension or a rubbery end point to extension indicates a positive bounce home test and is concerning for a meniscus tear or some other intra-articular pathology that provides a mechanical block to extension [3].

The Finochietto test or jump sign can be used to aid in the detection of tears of the posterior horn of the meniscus. To perform this test, an anterior translational force is applied to the proximal tibia, similar to the anterior drawer and Lachman tests, while the knee is held in 130–140° of flexion. This test is positive when the examiner

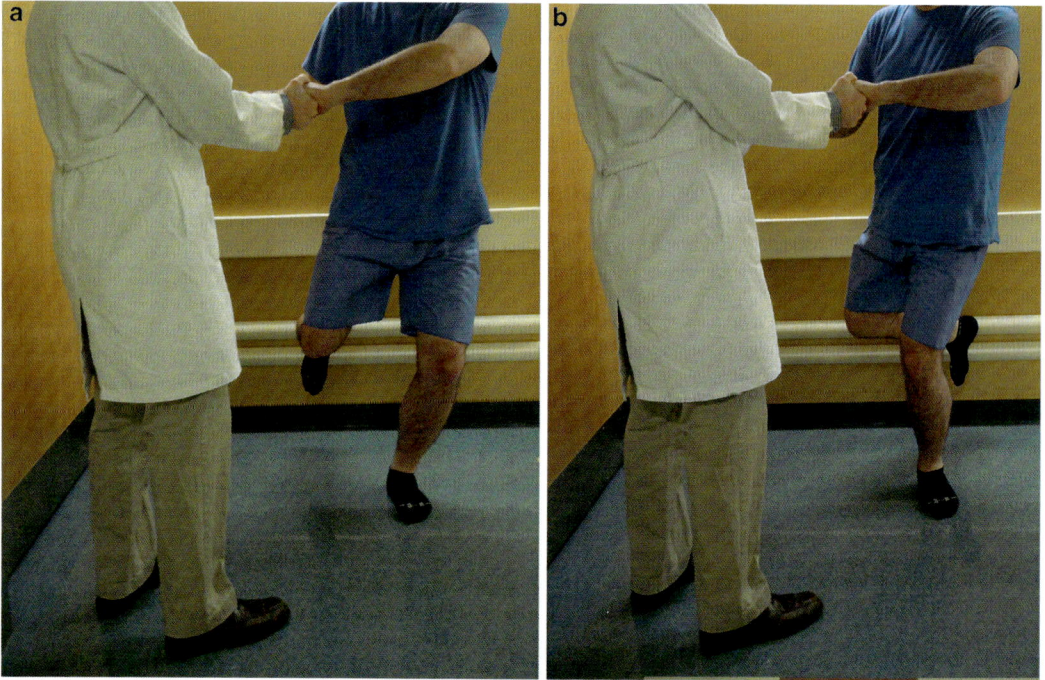

Fig. 2.4 Positioning for Thessaly test. (**a**) Thessaly test with external rotation of body. (**b**) Thessaly test with internal rotation of body

feels a "jump" when a torn posterior horn of the meniscus is displaced anterior to the tibiofemoral contact point [2].

The Boehler and Payr tests utilize the meniscal compression caused by varus and valgus stress testing to diagnose meniscus injuries. To perform the Boehler test, the examiner applies a varus force to compress the medial meniscus or a valgus force to compress the lateral meniscus with the knee in almost full extension. A positive test results from pain on the side of compression with this maneuver and is suggestive of meniscus injury, particularly in the anterior to middle section of the meniscus. The Payr test is similarly used to evaluate for medial meniscus tears by applying a varus force to compress the medial meniscus with the knee held in 90° of flexion [10].

The Thessaly and Childress tests are standing physical exam maneuvers that can aid in the detection of meniscus injury. These tests utilize the combination of axial load applied to the knee from standing to the rotational forces from designated maneuvers during the tests to elicit pain due to a meniscus tear. To perform the Thessaly test, the patient is asked to stand flat-footed with all weight on one extremity. While holding the examiner's hands for support, the patient is then asked to internally and externally rotate his or her knee and body three times while keeping the foot planted with the knee flexed at 5° and then with 20° of knee flexion (Fig. 2.4). The maneuver should first be performed on the patient's uninjured extremity prior to the symptomatic extremity to educate the patient on the physical exam technique. A positive result is indicated by medial or lateral joint-line pain with this maneuver and is concerning for meniscus injury [25]. When the Thessaly test is performed at 20° of knee flexion, it has been shown to have a high sensitivity for the detection of both medial and lateral meniscus tears (89 % and 92 %, respectively) [25]. The 20° Thessaly test also has been reported to have high specificity rates, 97 % and 96 %, for the detection of medial and lateral meniscus tears, respectively [25]. This test has a lower sensitivity and specificity when performed at 5° of knee flexion.

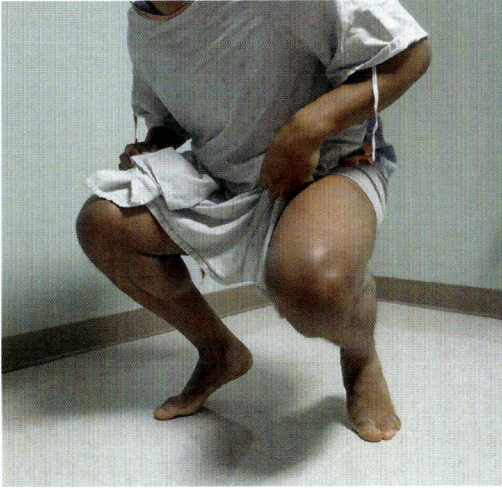

Fig. 2.5 Positioning for Childress test

The Childress test is performed by asking the patient to perform a "duck walk" by moving forward while maintaining full knee flexion (Fig. 2.5). Similar to the Thessaly test, this test is also positive for meniscal injury when the maneuver reproduces medial or lateral joint-line pain [10]. The Childress maneuver applies considerable compressive forces to the menisci and should not be performed in patients with a known positive McMurray test.

Conclusion

Due to the common occurrence of meniscus injuries, physicians should often consider the menisci as a potential source of knee pain and must be capable of performing a focused examination to aid in the diagnosis of a meniscus tear. While imaging techniques play an important role in confirming the diagnosis of meniscus injury, clinicians must utilize their physical examination skills to determine when obtaining advanced imaging is necessary. Understanding the physical examination of the knee, particularly relating to the meniscus, is essential for all practitioners responsible for caring for patients with knee pain. While the exhaustive use of all maneuvers is likely unnecessary to arrive at an accurate diagnosis, clinicians should be encouraged to become facile with 2 or 3 tests that are easily reproducible and can be applied to all patients presenting with knee pain. In this way, an individual examiner's sensitivity and specificity for detecting meniscal pathology will be optimized.

References

1. Poehling GG, Ruch DS, Chabon SJ. The landscape of meniscal injuries. Clin Sports Med. 1990;9:539–49.
2. Finochietto R. Semilunar cartilages of the knee: the "Jump Sign". J Bone Joint Surg. 1935;17(4):916–21.
3. Hoppenfeld S. Physical examination of the spine & extremities. Upper Saddle River, NJ: Prentice Hall; 1976.
4. Worsley P, Stokes M, Taylor M. Predicted knee kinematics and kinetics during functional activities using motion capture and musculoskeletal modeling in healthy older people. Gait Posture. 2011;33: 268–73.
5. Metcalf MH, Barrett GR. Prospective evaluation of 1485 meniscal tear patterns in patients with stable knees. Am J Sports Med. 2004;32:675–80.
6. Miller MD, Thompson SR, Hart JA. Review of orthopaedics. 6th ed. Philadelphia, PA: Elsevier; 2012.
7. Mayo Robson AW. Ruptured crucial ligaments and their repair by operation. Ann Surg. 1903;70:716–8.
8. Schraeder TL, Terek RM, Smith CC. Clinical evaluation of the knee. N Eng J Med. 2010;363(4):e5.
9. Malanga GA, Andrus S, Nadler SF, McLean J. Physical examination of the knee: A review of the original test description and scientific validity of common orthopedic tests. Arch Phys Med Rehabil. 2003; 84:592–603.
10. Shrier I, Boudier-Reveret M, Fahmy K. Understanding the different physical examination tests for suspected meniscal tears. Curr Sports Med Rep. 2010;9(5): 284–9.
11. Canale ST, Beaty JH. Acute traumatic lesions of ligaments in Campbell's Operative Orthopaedics. 11th ed. Philadelphia, PA: Elsevier; 2008.
12. Donaldson III WF, Warren RF, Wickiewicz T. A comparison of acute anterior cruciate ligament examinations. Initial versus examination under anesthesia. Am J Sports Med. 1985;13:5–10.
13. Jonsson T, Althoff B, Peterson L, Renstrom P. Clinical diagnosis of ruptures of the anterior drawer ligament: a comparative study of the Lachman test and the anterior drawer sign. Am J Sports Med. 1982;10:100–2.
14. Katz JW, Fingeroth RJ. The diagnostic accuracy of ruptures of the anterior cruciate ligament comparing the Lachman test, the anterior drawer sign, and the pivot shift test in acute and chronic knee injuries. Am J Sports Med. 1986;14:88–91.
15. Kim SJ, Kim HK. Reliability of the anterior drawer test, the pivot shift test, and the Lachman test. Clin Orthop. 1995;317:237–42.
16. Mitsou A, Vallianatos P. Clinical diagnosis of ruptures of the anterior cruciate ligament: comparison between

the Lachman test and the anterior drawer sign. Injury. 1988;18:427–8.

17. Torg JS, Conrad W, Kalen V. Clinical diagnosis of anterior cruciate ligament instability in the athlete. Am J Sports Med. 1976;4:84–93.

18. Galway HR, MacIntosh DL. The lateral pivot shift: a symptom and sign of anterior cruciate ligament insufficiency. Clin Orthop. 1980;147:45–50.

19. Rubinstein RA, Shelbourne KD, McCarroll JR, VanMeter CD, Rettig AC. The accuracy of the clinical examination in the setting of posterior cruciate ligament injuries. Am J Sports Med. 1994;22:550–7.

20. Daniel DM, Stone ML, Barnett P, Sachs R. Use of the quadriceps active test to diagnose posterior cruciate-ligament disruption and measure posterior laxity of the knee. J Bone Joint Surg Am. 1988;70:386–91.

21. Anderson AF, Lipscomb AB. Clinical diagnosis of meniscal tears. Description of a new manipulative test. Am J Sports Med. 1986;14:291–3.

22. Fowler PJ, Lubliner JA. The predictive value of five clinical signs in the evaluation of meniscal pathology. Arthroscopy. 1989;5:184–6.

23. Kurosaka M, Yagi M, Yoshiya S, Muratsu H, Mizuno K. Efficacy of the axially loaded pivot shift test for the diagnosis of a meniscal tear. Int Orthop. 1999;23: 271–4.

24. Evans PJ, Bell GD, Frank C. Prospective evaluation of the McMurray test. Am J Sport Med. 1993;21:604–8.

25. Karachalios T, Hantes M, Zibis AH, Zachos V, Karantanas AH, Malizos KN. Diagnostic accuracy of a new clinical test (the Thessaly test) for early detection of meniscal tears. J Bone Joint Surg. 2005;87(5): 955–62.

26. McMurray TP. The semilunar cartilages. Br J Surg. 1942;2(116):407–14.

27. Apley AG. The diagnosis of meniscus injuries: some new clinical methods. J Bone Joint Surg. 1947;29(1): 78–84.

Imaging of Meniscus Pathology

Nicole S. Belkin, Pramod B. Voleti, John D. Kelly IV, and Viviane Khoury

Introduction

Multiple systematic reviews of the literature aimed at determining the diagnostic value of physical examination maneuvers in the diagnosis of meniscal pathology have been conducted. Although studies have concluded a wide range in sensitivity and specificity, joint line tenderness can generally be considered a highly sensitive though nonspecific test. The McMurray and Apley tests can be considered less sensitive but more specific [1–3]. More recently described, the Thessaly test is reported to detect meniscal tears with a sensitivity of 90 % and a specificity of 98 % [4]. The predictive value of these maneuvers is further complicated by the practitioner's learning curve associated with detecting a positive finding and patient factors such as concomitant injury or secondary gain. Thus, no single clinical test, or combination thereof, can definitively establish a correct diagnosis of meniscal tear. Therefore, in the case of suspected meniscal injury, it is appropriate to obtain proper diagnostic imaging.

N.S. Belkin, M.D. (✉) • P.B. Voleti, M.D.
J.D. Kelly IV, M.D.
Department of Orthopaedic Surgery, Hospital of the University of Pennsylvania, 3400 Spruce Street, 2 Silverstein, Philadelphia, PA 19104, USA
e-mail: Nicole.belkin@uphs.epenn.edu

V. Khoury, M.D.
Department of Radiology, University of Pennsylvania, Philadelphia, PA, USA

Roentgenographic Evaluation

Radiographs are often overlooked in the setting of clinical concern for meniscal injury, but there are certain scenarios that warrant this assessment. For a patient with a history of injury, anteroposterior (AP) and lateral radiographs should be obtained to evaluate for possible fracture. In patients without a definitive mechanism of injury, radiographs should also be obtained to assess for an arthropathy or other osseous abnormality of the knee. In the setting of arthrosis, weight-bearing views should be obtained in addition to the AP and lateral views, as they provide a more accurate assessment of the degree of joint space narrowing of the medial and lateral tibiofemoral compartments. These views include weight-bearing AP views of both knees, as well as Rosenberg views (posteroanterior [PA], 45° flexion, weight-bearing views that are more sensitive and specific view for mild joint space narrowing) [5]. Patellofemoral joint space narrowing may be assessed on axial views of the patella in varying degrees of flexion, namely, skyline, Merchant, or sunrise views.

The presence of marginal osteophytes has a sensitivity of 83 % and a specificity of 93 % for the presence of osteoarthritis (OA) [6]. Prove et al. demonstrated that the medial tibiofemoral joint space is unchanged compared to preoperative images obtained in meniscectomized patients, suggesting that joint space narrowing is not a result of meniscal pathology, but rather pathognomonic for OA [7]. Radiologists suggest that subtle joint space narrowing may also be due exclusively to meniscal pathology. Rosenberg views are especially helpful when assessing the lateral compartment where degenerative changes appear to be more pronounced in early flexion (flexion gap disease) as opposed to the medial compartment where "extension gap" wear is more prevalent. Given the uncertainties associated with physical examination and radiographs, the definitive diagnosis of a meniscal tear is often made via advanced imaging modalities.

Magnetic Resonance Imaging

The primary imaging modality for the evaluation of intra-articular pathology of the knee is magnetic resonance imaging (MRI). MRI has been shown to have a sensitivity of 93 % and a specificity of 88 % for medial meniscus tears and a sensitivity of 79 % and a specificity of 95 % for lateral meniscus tears [8, 9].

Imaging Technique

A dedicated knee coil is utilized to provide an optimal signal-to-noise ratio. Axial, sagittal, and coronal sequences should be obtained with a slice thickness of no greater than 3 mm over a small (no greater than 16 cm) field of view. The sequences with the greatest sensitivity for the detection of meniscal tears are conventional spin-echo T1-weighted, proton density-weighted, and gradient-echo images [10]. T2-weighted images are associated with a lower sensitivity but a higher specificity and are therefore valuable for the confirmation of the presence of a tear visualized on one of the more sensitive sequences.

1.5 Versus 3.0 Tesla MRI

Prompted by advancements in imaging technology, there have been a few investigations into differential diagnostic accuracy between images acquired with different strength magnets. A number of groups have reported comparable sensitivity and specificity of 3T and 1.5T MRI for the diagnosis of meniscal tears with trends toward enhanced accuracy with 3T technology [11–13]. Furthermore, similar rates and causes of false-positive and false-negative diagnoses were found in those studies [11–13].

Although MRI at 3T has been shown to have better sensitivity and grading of cartilage lesions in the knee [15], it has not yet been shown to increase sensitivity or specificity of meniscal tears compared with 1.5T [12].

Normal Meniscal Appearance

Normal meniscus has uniformly low signal intensity on both T1- and T2-weighted images. In the sagittal plane, at the periphery of the tibiofemoral joint, the body of the meniscus is visible as a continuous, homogenous rectangle. Moving centrally, the anterior and posterior horns become visible as low-signal (black) triangles tapered inward, transiently resembling a bow tie, then distinctly separate at the roots. In the coronal plane anteriorly, the anterior horns and possibly the transverse (or intermeniscal) ligament are visible as somewhat rectangular in morphology. Moving posteriorly, the bodies become visible as low-signal triangles tapered centrally, and the posterior horns again have a rectangular morphology (Fig. 3.1).

Abnormal Meniscal Signals

A grading system exists for meniscal signal abnormalities. Higher grades are associated with more meniscal body involvement [14].

Grade 1 meniscal signals are focally increased signals that are globular in appearance and contained within the substance of the meniscus without coming into contact with the articular surface of the meniscus. These signals can be representative of mucinous and myxoid changes within the meniscus as a consequence of aging or areas of increased vascularity in children.

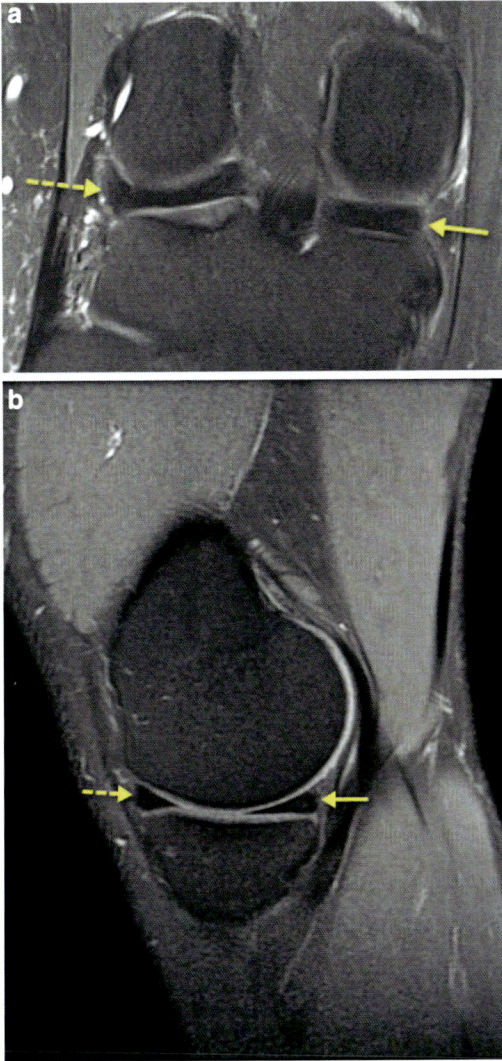

Fig. 3.1 Normal MRI appearance of menisci. (**a**) Coronal fat-saturated proton density-weighted sequence showing the normal, hypointense, and rectangular appearance of the posterior horns of the medial (*arrow*) and lateral meniscus (*dashed arrow*) in the coronal plane. (**b**) Sagittal fat-saturated proton density-weighted sequence showing the normal, hypointense, triangular appearance of the anterior (*arrow*) and posterior horn (*dashed arrow*) of the medial meniscus

Grade 2 meniscal signals are linear regions of increased signal intensity that also do not extend to the articular surface of the meniscus. These signals are believed to be associated with meniscal degeneration, representing disruption of the normal collagen orientation.

Grade 3 meniscal signals are globular, linear, or complex areas of increased signal that extend to at least one articular surface. In the setting of grade 3 signal visualization on MRI, tears are identifiable arthroscopically in greater than 90 % of cases [16, 17]. Additionally, grade 3 signals can serve to heighten the index of suspicion for a closed meniscal tear and assist in the surgeon's ability to identify these lesions via arthroscopic probing.

Classification of Meniscal Tears

The two primary criteria for the diagnosis of meniscal tears are intrameniscal signal that contacts the superior and/or inferior articular surface and/or abnormal meniscal morphology [8].

A commonly used classification of meniscal tears includes the following types: longitudinal, radial, displaced flap, bucket-handle, and complex.

Longitudinal tears, the most frequent type, are classified as horizontal (dividing the meniscus into an upper and lower segment), or vertical (dividing the meniscus into an inner and outer segment).

Longitudinal horizontal tears, also known as cleavage tears, are oriented parallel to or at a slight angle relative to the joint surface and perpendicular to the meniscocapsular junction (Fig. 3.2). Longitudinal horizontal tears are often associated with mucoid degeneration, and the associated signals may be difficult to distinguish on MRI (Fig. 3.3).

Longitudinal vertical tears are oriented perpendicular to the joint surface (Fig. 3.4). The etiology of these tears is commonly acute injury.

When the portion of the meniscus central to a longitudinal tear becomes displaced or "flips" into the intercondylar notch, this is referred to as a "bucket-handle" tear [10] (Fig. 3.5).

Radial tears extend from the central portion of the meniscus radially outward toward the periphery and may be partial or full thickness (Fig. 3.6). These tears are oriented perpendicular to the longitudinal collagen bundles of the meniscus [20]. Such tears sometimes extend anterolaterally or

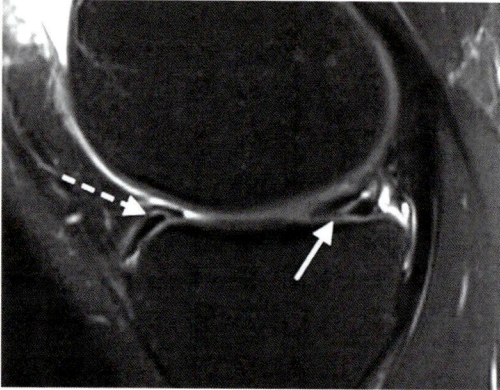

Fig. 3.2 Posterior horn horizontal tear. Sagittal fat-saturated T2-weighted image in a 39-year-old male shows linear internal meniscal signal contacting inferior medial meniscal surface (*arrow*). Note normal transverse (intermeniscal) ligament (*dashed arrow*) associated with the normal anterior horn, not to be confused with a meniscal tear

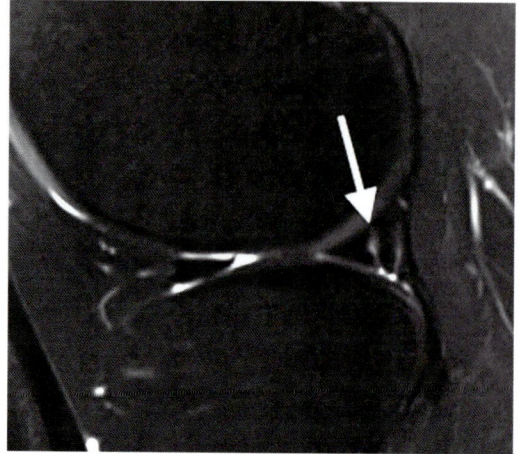

Fig. 3.4 Peripheral longitudinal vertical tear of posterior horn. Sagittal fat-saturated proton density image in a 27-year-old male shows a peripheral vertical signal within the posterior horn of the lateral meniscus (*arrow*) representing a tear

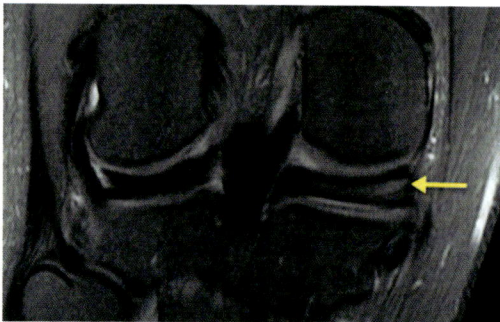

Fig. 3.3 Mucoid changes versus longitudinal horizontal tear. Coronal fat-saturated proton density-weighted image in a 41-year-old male shows abnormal horizontal signal (*arrow*) in the posterior horn of the medial meniscus, which may represent myxoid degenerative changes and/or a longitudinal horizontal meniscal tear

posterolaterally and are then referred to as parrot-beak or flap tears. Radial and flap tears account for approximately 5–10 % of meniscal tears.

A meniscal fragment may become displaced away from the site of tear, referred to as a *displaced flap* tear. Patients may present with locking in addition to knee pain. Like a radial tear, a displaced flap tear is manifested by a truncated or shortened appearance, but with a meniscal fragment that is typically flipped peripherally (Fig. 3.7).

Complex tears contain tears in multiple planes, typically with extensive morphological changes of the meniscus including loss of substance (Fig. 3.8).

Another important type of meniscal tear is the root ligament tear or avulsion. Disruption of the root ligament of a meniscus disrupts the hoop tension and load distribution function of the meniscus [21]. The most common root tears occur in the posterior horn of the medial meniscus, typically representing a degenerative type of tear (Fig. 3.9a). Loss of the posterior anchor allows the meniscus to extrude medially and become less effective at shock dissipation.

A tear that occurs in the peripheral third of the meniscus may heal spontaneously or be successfully repaired, due to the vascular nature of this portion of the meniscus [18].

Associated and Secondary Signs of Meniscal Tears

Meniscal cysts are frequently associated with meniscal tears [22]. A meniscal (or intrameniscal) cyst is defined as a focus of high signal within a swollen meniscus. In the setting of increased pressure, fluid from an intrameniscal cyst can be

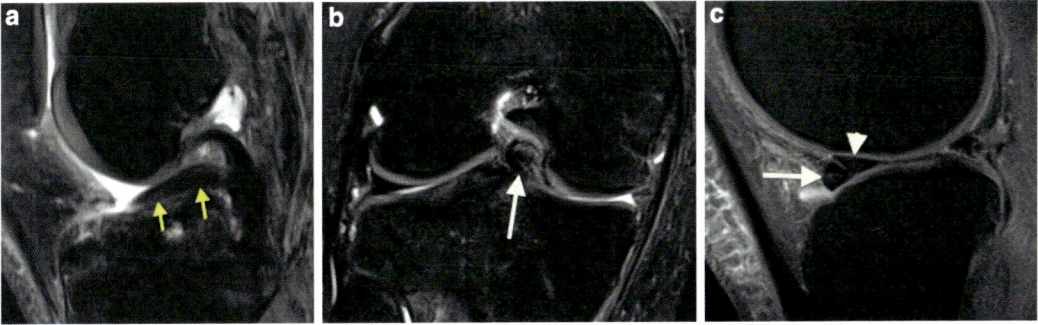

Fig. 3.5 Bucket-handle tears. Bucket-handle tear of the medial meniscus in a 25-year-old male with a large central meniscal fragment, seen on sagittal fat-saturated T2-weighted image (**a**) ("double PCL sign," *arrows*) and on coronal fat-saturated proton density image (**b**) (*arrow*). (**c**) Bucket-handle tear of lateral meniscus in a 20-year-old male seen on sagittal fat-saturated proton density image as a fragment flipped interiorly (*arrowhead*), abutting the anterior horn (*arrow*) ("flipped meniscus sign")

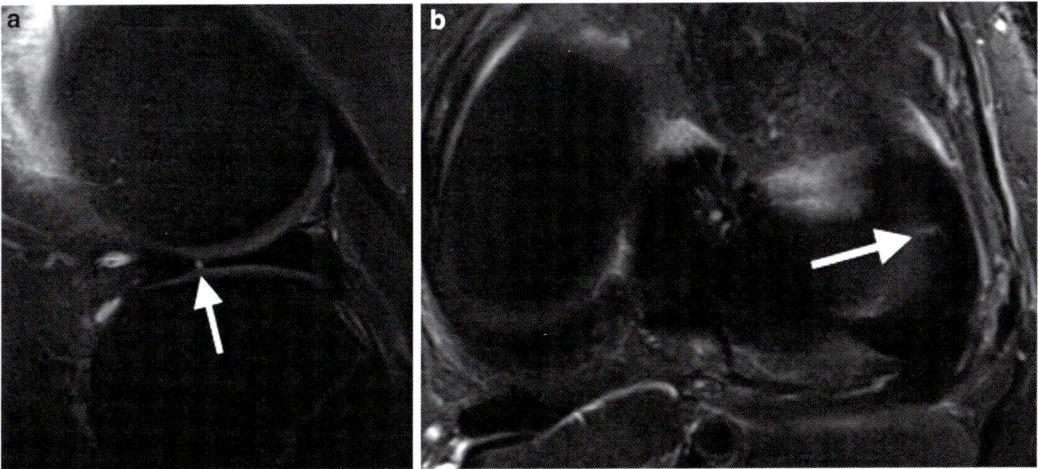

Fig. 3.6 Radial tear at junction of body and anterior horn. Sagittal fat-saturated T2-weighted image (**a**) and axial fat-saturated proton density image (**b**) in a 20-year-old male shows a fine linear fluid cleft (*arrows*), typical for a partial radial tear

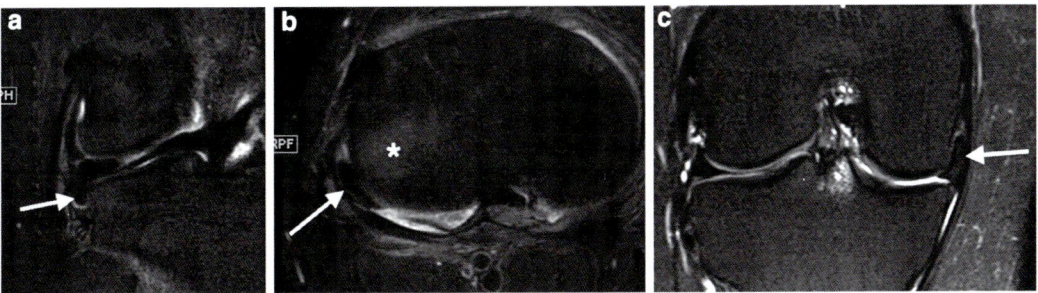

Fig. 3.7 Displaced flap tears lateral meniscal flap in popliteal hiatus in a 15-year-old male, on coronal fat-saturated T2-weighted image (**a**) and on axial fat-saturated proton density-weighted image (**b**) (*arrows*). Note reactive marrow edema of the adjacent tibia in B (*asterisk*). (**c**) Medial meniscal flap in a 53-year-old male seen on coronal fat-saturated proton density-weighted image, with blunting of the free inner margin of the body of the medial meniscus (*arrow*), with an associated inferior flap component in the medial gutter (between MCL and tibia) (*dashed arrow*)

squeezed or extravasated into the surrounding peripheral soft tissues, forming a parameniscal (also known as a perimeniscal) cyst [23]. Horizontal tears are also commonly associated with intra- or parameniscal cysts, as their orientation allows for synovial fluid extravasation

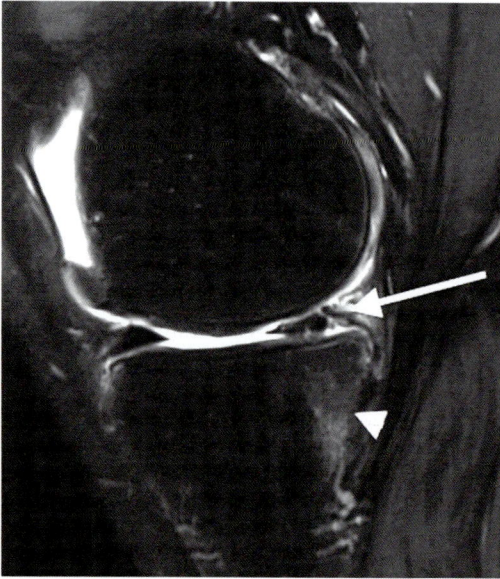

Fig. 3.8 Complex tear. Sagittal proton density image in a 66-year-old male shows a complex pattern of abnormal signal as well as morphological distortion of the posterior horn of the medial meniscus. Note reactive marrow edema of the adjacent tibia (*arrowhead*)

through the tear but then acts as a one-way valve (Fig. 3.10) [19].

Although laterally located cysts are more easily detectable clinically and potentially more symptomatic, the incidence of medial- and lateral-sided cysts is similar [24].

Meniscal extrusion (visualization of meniscal tissue that extends peripherally beyond the tibial margin) may be associated with meniscal root tears (Fig. 3.9b) but, importantly, may also be found in the setting of cartilage loss without a meniscal tear. Meniscal extrusion typically occurs in the setting of a meniscal root tear or may result from a meniscal tear with significant disruption of the circumferential collagen fibers. Occasionally, meniscal extrusion is seen with advanced cartilage disease of the respective compartment. Meniscal extrusion has been found to be strongly associated with the development or progression of osteoarthritis [25, 26].

Bone marrow edema adjacent to the meniscus, linear or diffuse, has also been shown to be highly indicative of meniscal tear (see Fig. 3.8). Bergin et al. sought to determine the frequency of abnormal MR signal intensity in soft tissues and osseous structures in association with surgically proven meniscal tears [7]. In addition to describing the high positive predictive values of the aforementioned meniscal cysts, meniscal extrusion, and bone marrow edema, they also

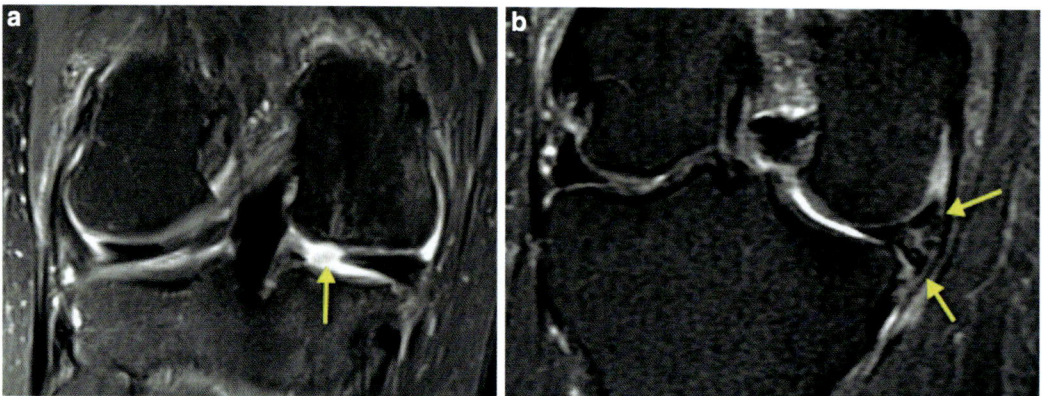

Fig. 3.9 Root ligament avulsions. (**a**) Coronal fat-saturated proton density-weighted image in a 50-year-old male shows a large tear of the root ligament of the posterior horn of the medial meniscus. (**b**) Peripheral extrusion of the body of the medial meniscus with a complex tear (*arrows*) in a 69-year-old female who also had a posterior root ligament tear (not shown)

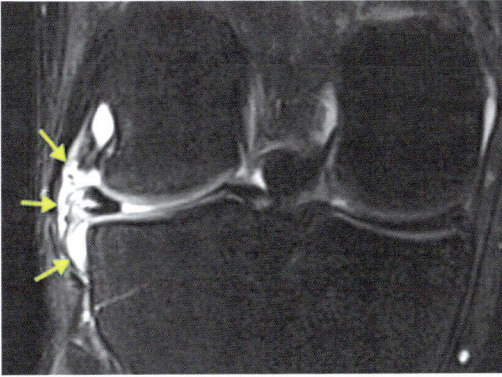

Fig. 3.10 Parameniscal cyst. Coronal fat-saturated proton density-weighted image in a 26-year-old male shows a lobulated parameniscal cyst (*arrows*) associated with a horizontal tear of the body of the lateral meniscus

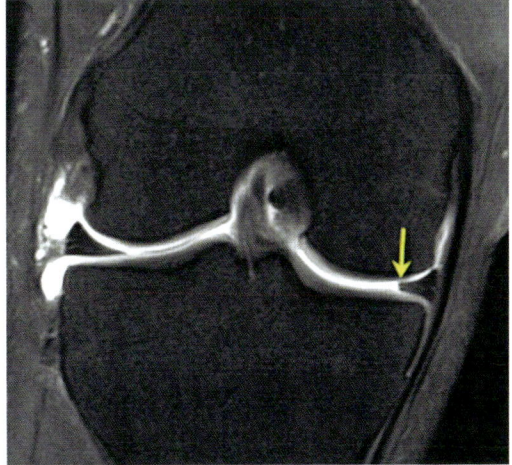

Fig. 3.11 MR arthrogram post meniscectomy. Coronal fat-saturated T1-weighted image post intra-articular gadolinium injection in a 19-year-old male shows blunting of the body of the medial meniscus (*arrow*), a typical appearance post partial meniscectomy. There is no gadolinium contrast (*bright signal*) within the meniscus to suggest a re-tear or residual tear

characterized the diagnostic value of the findings of cartilage loss near the meniscus, signal changes or edema about the MCL, effusion, and perimeniscal edema [27].

False-Positive Diagnosis

There are a number of normal anatomic structures, variants, and conditions that can lead to the false-positive diagnosis of meniscal tear. These include, but are not limited to, the transverse intermeniscal ligament (anterior horn tear) (see Fig. 3.2), the popliteus tendon (lateral meniscus tear), meniscofemoral ligaments, oblique meniscomeniscal ligament, chondrocalcinosis, and healed tears [28].

Repairability as Predicted by MRI

Nourissat et al. sought to describe criteria predictive of a surgeon's ability to repair a meniscus tear based upon MR imaging [29]. They described MRI criteria that include visualization of a rim of meniscal tissue 4 mm or less and presence of a longitudinally oriented lesion 10 mm or greater that could predict the reparability of the meniscus tear. They concluded that longitudinal full-thickness meniscus lesions are an indication for

repair in young active patients when located in red–red or red–white zones.

Magnetic Resonance Arthrography

There are pitfalls in applying the classic MR criteria of meniscal tears in the assessment of menisci following partial meniscectomies. Persistent increased surfacing intrameniscal (grade 3) signal intensity, a standard MR imaging criterion for meniscal tear, is frequently found in patients despite arthroscopic or clinical evidence of meniscal healing [30]. The finding is indicative of possible reparative fibrovascular scar tissue at the site of incompletely healed tears or of fluid at the site of recurrent residual tear.

Following meniscal repair, MR arthrography can serve as a useful tool in the diagnosis of reinjury or failure of repair [31–33]. Similarly, after previous partial meniscal resection, MR arthrography may provide slightly increased accuracy in detection of meniscal pathology when compared to un-enhanced magnetic resonance imaging when the resection involved <25 % of the meniscus (Fig. 3.11) [34].

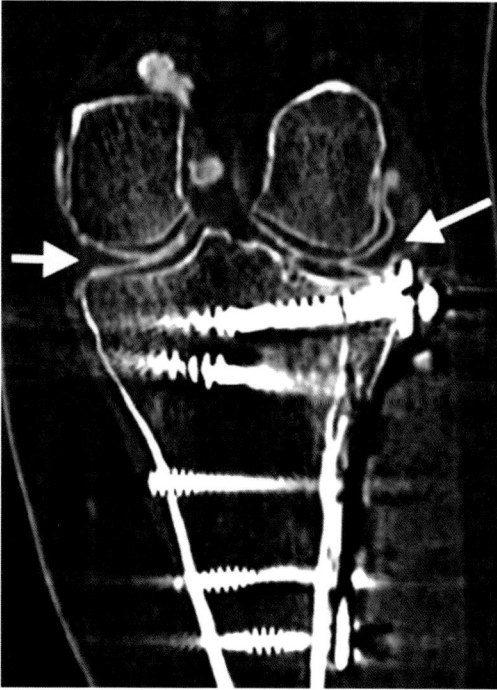

Fig. 3.12 CT arthrogram of the knee. Coronal refor-matted image post intra-articular iodinated contrast injec-tion. Both medial (*arrow*) and lateral (*dashed arrow*) menisci are well visualized as filling defects even with the presence of hardware in the tibia

Computed Tomography Arthrography

Computed tomography arthrography (CT arthrography) can be utilized in the diagnosis of meniscal pathology when the patient is not a candidate for MRI or in the event that adjacent orthopedic hardware that would diminish the quality of traditional MR images is present [35] (Fig. 3.12).

Ultrasound

Ultrasound (US) is of some but limited use in the diagnosis of meniscal pathology. Tears and extru-sion of the body of the meniscus can frequently be detected, but evaluation of the anterior and posterior horns is limited. US is also useful in the detection of perimeniscal cysts.

Summary

Due to the inaccuracies of physical examination and the deficiencies of plain radiographs, the role of MRI imaging has become increasingly impor-tant in the diagnosis of meniscal injury. Certain tear patterns have distinctive MRI appearances which may facilitate timely diagnosis.

References

1. Ryzewicz M, Peterson B, Siparsky PN, Bartz RL. The diagnosis of meniscus tears: the role of MRI and clinical examination. Clin Orthop Relat Res. 2007; 455:123–33. Epub 2007/02/07.
2. Scholten RJ, Deville WL, Opstelten W, Bijl D, van der Plas CG, Bouter LM. The accuracy of physical diagnostic tests for assessing meniscal lesions of the knee: a meta-analysis. J Fam Pract. 2001;50(11): 938–44. Epub 2001/11/17.
3. Solomon DH, Simel DL, Bates DW, Katz JN, Schaffer JL. The rational clinical examination. Does this patient have a torn meniscus or ligament of the knee? Value of the physical examination. JAMA. 2001; 286(13):1610–20.
4. Harrison BK, Abell BE, Gibson TW. The Thessaly test for detection of meniscal tears: validation of a new physical examination technique for primary care medicine. Clin J Sport Med. 2009;19(1):9–12. Epub 2009/01/07.
5. Rosenberg TD, Paulos LE, Parker RD, Coward DB, Scott SM. The forty-five-degree posteroanterior flexion weight-bearing radiograph of the knee. J Bone Joint Surg Am. 1988;70(10):1479–83. Epub 1988/12/01.
6. Altman R, Asch E, Bloch D, Bole G, Borenstein D, Brandt K, et al. Development of criteria for the classification and reporting of osteoarthritis. Classi-fication of osteoarthritis of the knee. Diagnostic and Therapeutic Criteria Committee of the American Rheumatism Association. Arthritis Rheum. 1986; 29(8):1039–49. Epub 1986/08/01.
7. Prove S, Charrois O, Dekeuwer P, Fallet L, Beaufils P. Comparison of the medial femorotibial joint space before and immediately after meniscectomy. Rev Chir Orthop Reparatrice Appar Mot. 2004;90(7):636–42. Epub 2004/12/31. Hauteur radiologique de l'interligne femoro-tibial medial avant et immediatement apres meniscectomie.
8. Manaster BJ. Magnetic resonance imaging of the knee. Semin Ultrasound CT MR. 1990;11:307–26.
9. Oei EH, Nikken JJ, Verstijnen AC, Ginai AZ, Myriam Hunink MG. MR imaging of the menisci and cruciate ligaments: a systematic review. Radiology. 2003; 226(3):837–48. Epub 2003/02/26.

10. Helms CA. The meniscus: recent advances in MR imaging of the knee. AJR Am J Roentgenol. 2002; 179(5):1115–22. Epub 2002/10/22.

11. Magee T, Williams D. 3.0-T MRI of meniscal tears. Am J Roentgenol. 2006;187(2):371–5.

12. Grossman JW, De Smet AA, Shinki K. Comparison of the accuracy rates of 3-T and 1.5-T MRI of the knee in the diagnosis of meniscal tear. AJR. Am J Roentgenol. 2009;193(2):509–14.

13. Van Dyck P, Vanhoenacker FM, Gielen JL, Dossche L, Weyler J, Parizel PM. Three-Tesla magnetic resonance imaging of the meniscus of the knee: What about equivocal errors? Acta Radiol. 2010;51(3): 296–301. Epub 2010/01/29.

14. Stoller DW, Martin C, Crues III JV, Kaplan L, Mink JH. Meniscal tears: pathologic correlation with MR imaging. Radiology. 1987;163(3):731–5.

15. Wong S, Steinbach L, Zhao J, Stehling C, Ma CB, Link TM. Comparative study of imaging at 3.0 T versus 1.5 T of the knee. Skeletal Radiol. 2009;38(8):761–9.

16. Crues 3rd JV, Mink J, Levy TL, Lotysch M, Stoller DW. Meniscal tears of the knee: accuracy of MR imaging. Radiology. 1987;164(2):445–8. Epub 1987/08/01.

17. Kaplan PA, Nelson NL, Garvin KL, Brown DE. MR of the knee: the significance of high signal in the meniscus that does not clearly extend to the surface. AJR Am J Roentgenol. 1991;156(2):333–6. Epub 1991/02/01.

18. Rubin DA, Kneeland JB, Listerud J, Underberg-Davis SJ, Dalinka MK. MR diagnosis of meniscal tears of the knee: value of fast spin-echo vs conventional spin-echo pulse sequences. AJR Am J Roentgenol. 1994;162(5):1131–5. Epub 1994/05/01.

19. Burk Jr DL, Dalinka MK, Kanal E, Schiebler ML, Cohen EK, Prorok RJ, et al. Meniscal and ganglion cysts of the knee: MR evaluation. AJR Am J Roentgenol. 1988;150(2):331–6. Epub 1988/02/01.

20. Tuckman GA, Miller WJ, Remo JW, Fritts HM, Rozansky MI. Radial tears of the menisci: MR findings. AJR Am J Roentgenol. 1994;163(2):395–400. Epub 1994/08/01.

21. Petersen W, Tillmann B. Collagenous fibril texture of the human knee joint menisci. Anat Embryol. 1998;197(4):317–24. Epub 1998/06/13.

22. Campbell SE, Sanders TG, Morrison WB. MR imaging of meniscal cysts: incidence, location, and clinical significance. AJR Am J Roentgenol. 2001; 177(2):409–13. Epub 2001/07/20.

23. Helms CA, Laorr A, Cannon Jr WD. The absent bow tie sign in bucket-handle tears of the menisci in the knee. AJR Am J Roentgenol. 1998;170(1):57–61. Epub 1998/01/10.

24. Tasker AD, Ostlere SJ. Relative incidence and morphology of lateral and medial meniscal cysts detected by magnetic resonance imaging. Clin Radiol. 1995; 50(11):778–81. Epub 1995/11/01.

25. Costa CR, Morrison WB, Carrino JA. Medial meniscus extrusion on knee MRI: is extent associated with severity of degeneration or type of tear? AJR Am J Roentgenol. 2004;183(1):17–23. Epub 2004/06/23.

26. Lerer DB, Umans HR, Hu MX, Jones MH. The role of meniscal root pathology and radial meniscal tear in medial meniscal extrusion. Skeletal Radiol. 2004; 33(10):569–74. Epub 2004/08/19.

27. Bergin D, Hochberg H, Zoga AC, Qazi N, Parker L, Morrison WB. Indirect soft-tissue and osseous signs on knee MRI of surgically proven meniscal tears. AJR Am J Roentgenol. 2008;191(1):86–92. Epub 2008/06/20.

28. De Smet AA, Norris MA, Yandow DR, Graf BK, Keene JS. Diagnosis of meniscal tears of the knee with MR imaging: effect of observer variation and sample size on sensitivity and specificity. AJR Am J Roentgenol. 1993;160(3):555–9. Epub 1993/03/01.

29. Nourissat G, Beaufils P, Charrois O, Selmi TA, Thoreux P, Moyen B, et al. Magnetic resonance imaging as a tool to predict reparability of longitudinal full-thickness meniscus lesions. Knee Surg Sports Traumatol Arthrosc. 2008;16(5):482–6. Epub 2008/02/23.

30. Deutsch AL, Mink JH, Fox JM, Arnoczky SP, Rothman BJ, Stoller DW, et al. Peripheral meniscal tears: MR findings after conservative treatment or arthroscopic repair. Radiology. 1990;176(2):485–8. Epub 1990/08/01.

31. Toms AP, White LM, Marshall TJ, Donell ST. Imaging the post-operative meniscus. Eur J Radiol. 2005;54(2):189–98. Epub 2005/04/20.

32. Farley TE, Howell SM, Love KF, Wolfe RD, Neumann CH. Meniscal tears: MR and arthrographic findings after arthroscopic repair. Radiology. 1991;180(2): 517–22. Epub 1991/08/01.

33. Totty WG, Matava MJ. Imaging the postoperative meniscus. Magn Reson Imaging Clin N Am. 2000; 8(2):271–83. Epub 2000/07/06.

34. White LM, Schweitzer ME, Weishaupt D, Kramer J, Davis A, Marks PH. Diagnosis of recurrent meniscal tears: prospective evaluation of conventional MR imaging, indirect MR arthrography, and direct MR arthrography. Radiology. 2002;222(2):421–9. Epub 2002/01/31.

35. Malghem J, Vande berg BC, Lebon C, Lecouvet FE, Maldague BE. Ganglion cysts of the knee: articular communication revealed by delayed radiography and CT after arthrography. AJR Am J Roentgenol. 1998; 170(6):1579–83. Epub 1998/06/03.

Meniscectomy: The Basics

4

John G. Horneff III and John D. Kelly IV

Introduction

The menisci of the knee have a limited blood supply stemming from the superior and inferior medial and lateral geniculate arteries. The nutrient vessels that nourish the menisci enter from the periphery of knee near its capsule and taper off as they move towards the center of the knee. Miller, Warner, and Harner classified this tapering vascularity into three zones (from outside to inside): red, red–white, and white. Essentially, the meniscal tissue of the red zone has very good blood supply, which leaves tears in this region amenable to repair [1]. In contrast, tears seen in white zone and, to a lesser extent, the red–white zone are often irreparable. Since these tears cannot be repaired, arthroscopic partial meniscectomy has evolved to improve function, relieve pain, and preserve as much of the uninjured meniscus as possible. Partial meniscectomy is the most commonly performed orthopedic procedure in the USA. When properly performed, it can afford years of relief to most patients.

J.G. Horneff III, M.D. (✉) • J.D. Kelly IV, M.D.
Department of Orthopaedic Surgery,
Hospital of the University of Pennsylvania,
3400 Spruce Street, 2 Silverstein Building,
Floor 2, Philadelphia, PA 19104, USA
e-mail: John.horneff@uphs.upenn.edu

Indications

The indications for arthroscopic intervention of meniscal tears include the following: (1) symptoms of meniscal injury that affect activities of daily living, work, or sports (e.g., locking, instability, effusion, pain); (2) positive physical findings of joint line tenderness, joint effusion, limitations of motion, and positive provocative signs; (3) failure to respond to nonsurgical treatment; and (4) a ruling out of other pathology of knee pain identified in patient history, physical examination, or imaging studies. Patients identified to have one of these criteria are then further categorized into having tears that can be repaired versus those that must be excised.

Although all tears should be properly assessed during diagnostic arthroscopy before deciding whether repair or excision is performed, there are some general guidelines that often direct a surgeon to perform meniscectomy. The most important of these guidelines is the location of the tear in respect to the three zones of vascularity. Any tear found in the white zone has essentially no healing potential and should be excised. This includes radial, oblique, flap, horizontal cleavage, and complex tears. In contrast, tears found in the red–red zone that are vertical longitudinal in nature or bucket-handle tears that remain in good condition once they are reduced are amenable to repair. Red–white tears are indeed more controversial and may be repaired with a biologic augmentation technique. This will be discussed in subsequent chapters.

Regardless of the eventual surgical plan, any patient that is to undergo surgery should have a discussion that explains the risks and benefits of surgery, why removal versus repair is being chosen, and that recurrence is a possibility. Similarly, proper preoperative imaging (i.e. MRI) and clearance should always be performed to ensure that the proper surgery occurs in the safest possible fashion.

Goals

Metcalf et al. best defined the goals of arthroscopic partial meniscectomy in the 1990s. The general guidelines are as follows: (1) any mobile fragments that can be introduced past the inner margin of the meniscus at the center of the joint should be removed; (2) the remaining meniscal rim following excision should be smoothed to avoid any sudden changes in contour that might lead to further tearing; (3) a perfectly smooth rim is not necessary as repeat arthroscopy has shown rim remodeling and smoothing at 6–9 months; (4) the arthroscopic probe should be used repeatedly during the procedure to gain information about the mobility and texture of the remaining rim; (5) the meniscocapsular junction and the peripheral meniscal rim should be protected to maintain meniscal stability and preserve the load transmission properties of the meniscus; (6) to optimize efficiency, both manual and motorized resection instruments should be used. Manual instruments allow for more controlled resection, while motorized instruments remove loose debris and smooth frayed fragments; (7) in uncertain situations, more rather than less intact meniscal rim should be preserved to avoid segmental resection, which would essentially result in a total meniscectomy [2]. Respecting these guidelines allows for proper meniscal excision that also best preserves viable tissue.

Positioning

When performing partial meniscectomy, the correct positioning of the patient is paramount to visualizing all aspects of the knee joint anatomy

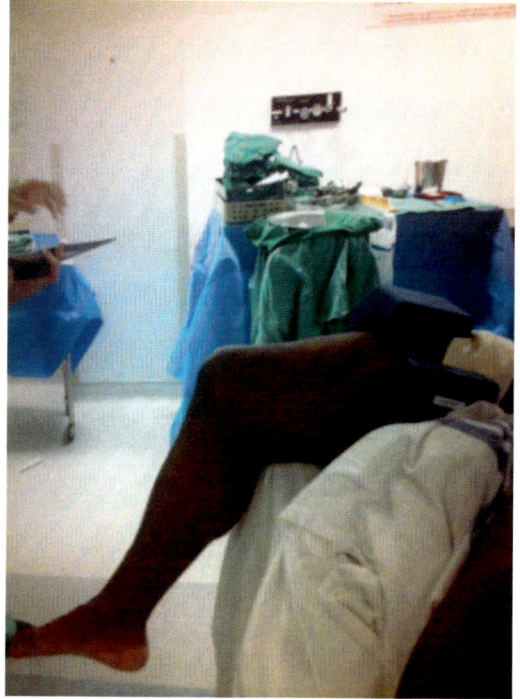

Fig. 4.1 Positioning of the operative leg in a standard circumferential leg holder proximal to the knee

and preventing damage to tissues. Typically, the patient is placed supine on a standard operating table. The operative leg must be able to hang over the side of the table during the operation so that the standard anteromedial and anterolateral portals can be created in a controlled and safe manner. To help with visualization of the medial compartment of the knee, a lateral (valgus) post is often attached to the bed about three to four fingerbreadths proximal to the level of the knee joint (Fig. 4.1). Alternatively, as the authors prefer, a commercial, well-padded leg holder facilitates access to tight compartments and affords extension and stretching of the posterior capsule. As the operative leg is brought over the side of the operating table, the force applied by the lateral post or leg holder on the thigh creates a valgus stress on the knee that opens the medial joint space of the knee, which can allow for better visualization and safer navigation (Fig. 4.2). When using this post, injury may occur to the medial collateral ligament (MCL). However, the senior author has not noticed any long-term sequelae of MCL stretching. In fact, for older,

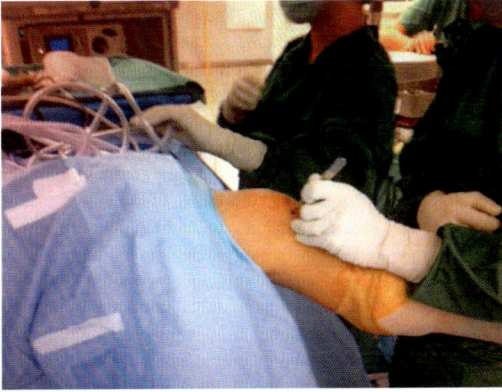

Fig. 4.2 A knee undergoing valgus stress which allows for opening and visualization of the medial compartment

more degenerative knees, the authors commonly surgically release the proximal MCL (see below) to gain access to the posterior horn.

Technique and Portal Placement

After appropriate positioning, prepping, and draping of the patient, the knee is typically examined under anesthesia. The purpose of this examination is to establish the anatomical landmarks of the knee and to assess any possible instability from ligamentous injury. Findings from examination should correlate with the arthroscopic findings—i.e. a suspected varus injury should be accompanied by increased visualization of the lateral compartment. Following examination, the knee is positioned over the side of the table for presurgical marking of the surface anatomy and arthroscopic portal placement. The soft tissue and bony landmarks of interest for the standard anteromedial and anterolateral portals include the following: the inferior border of the patella, the patellar tendon, and the tibial plateau.

The surgeon is best able to assess the edges of these structures by rolling a thumb or index finger along their borders. Once properly located, a marking pen is used to mark the inferomedial and inferolateral borders of the patella continuing down to the respective medial and lateral edges of the patellar tendon. Lastly, the edges of the medial and lateral tibial plateau are palpated and marked. Although not all surgeons will choose

to mark out these anatomical landmarks, doing so can prevent errant portal placement, injury to structures, and allow for proper adjustment to variations in patient anatomy. Next, the projected anteromedial and anterolateral portals can be marked.

There are various philosophies for choosing portal placement. A standard method is marking the anterolateral portal 1 cm off the lateral edge of the patellar tendon and the anteromedial portal 1.5 cm off the medial edge of the patellar tendon with both halfway between the inferior border of the patella and superior border of the tibial plateau. Another method is based on individual patient anatomy and involves feeling for the "soft spot" at the apex of "Joyce Hardy Triangle" which is bound by the patellar tendon, tibial plateau, and edge of the femoral condyle. The senior author ascribes to two basic arthroscopic principles: (1) look high, work low and (2) create portals in the position with which they will be employed. In a medial meniscectomy, for example, a high lateral portal is best created at the "vertex" of the junction of the lateral femoral condyle and the patella. This high placement allows the arthroscope to traverse the medial tibial spine and afford an excellent view of the posterior horn of the medial meniscus. A "low" working medial portal is created approximately 5 mm medial to the patella tendon and just above the joint surface (Fig. 4.3). A high lateral viewing portal also affords excellent instrument access to the posterior medial horn when the viewing portal is switched to the medial side. Both portals are created in slight flexion and valgus: the positions used for the procedure. Similarly, for a lateral meniscal resection, the leg is placed in a "figure of four" position on a padded Mayo stand, and a "high" medial viewing portal is created in the medial "vertex" of the junction of the patella and medial femoral condyle. A low lateral working portal is made under direct vision just lateral to the patella tendon at the joint line. Whichever method is chosen, it is important to remember that the anterolateral portal tends to be placed slightly higher than the anteromedial portal for medial meniscectomy. This accounts for the slightly higher border of the lateral tibial plateau compared to the medial plateau.

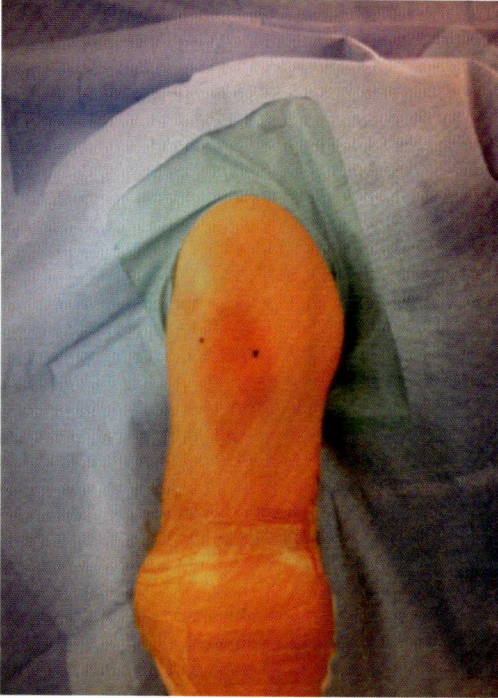

Fig. 4.3 Standard portal placement for knee arthroscopy with higher placement of the lateral portal compared to the medial portal

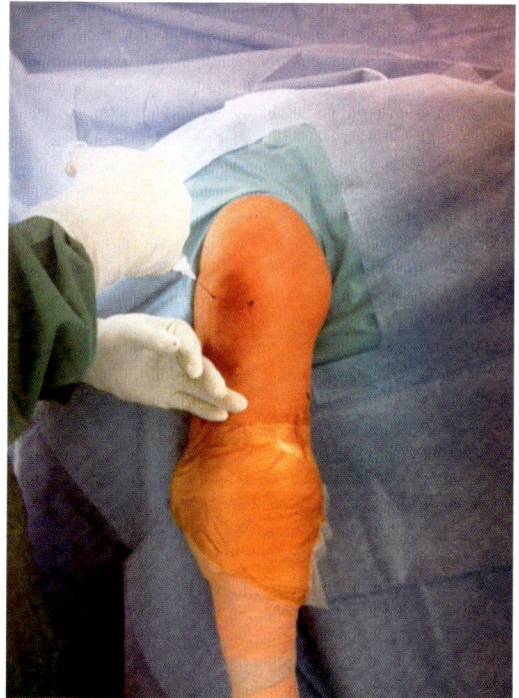

Fig. 4.4 Before incision, local anesthetic injection of the portal sites with epinephrine additive helps to decrease the bleeding caused by incisional wounds

After marking out the surface anatomy and projected portal sites, local anesthetic with epinephrine can be injected into the portal sites to help decrease the amount of capsular bleeding (Fig. 4.4). The use of a tourniquet is optional but is favored by the senior author to help decrease bleeding and subsequently increase visualization. An 11-blade is first used to create the anterolateral portal, which serves as the primary visualization portal. The blade is introduced into the skin in a vertical fashion with the bevel facing up to prevent inadvertent injury to the anterior horn of the meniscus. As the blade is passed through the skin, it is aimed towards the notch of the femur and continued about 1.5 cm deep to incise the capsule. This incision can then be dilated with the use of a hemostat introduced into the same path. The blunt trocar for the arthroscope is then introduced into the joint by first aiming towards the notch in the same pathway as the incision and then medially towards the medial compartment. Once in the medial hemijoint, the blunt trocar is removed from the cannulae, and the camera is introduced with saline inflow attached.

Typically, an entire knee arthroscopy can be performed using a 30° scope. The senior author favors the usage of the 2.9 mm sheath as it allows enhanced posterior access in tighter knees. This 30° objective allows for visualization of the majority of the knee and is certainly capable of helping perform basic meniscectomy. It is important to remember throughout the process of the knee arthroscopy that turning the objective prior to advancing the camera towards a certain region allows for better visualization. Much like one would turn their head in the direction they are heading prior towards walking in that direction, the use of the 30° objective allows for safe passage through the knee. With the scope placed in the anterolateral portal, the objective is turned to face medially to help with direct visual placement of the anteromedial portal. An 18-gauge spinal needle is placed at the site of the proposed anteromedial portal. The direct visualization from the arthroscope ensures that the anterior meniscus and articular surfaces are protected during portal creation. Once the spinal needle is placed in the proper projection into the knee, the 11-blade is then inserted in a vertical fashion with the bevel up directly along the path of the needle. At this point, the primary working antero-medial has been created and the surgical arthroscopy can begin.

Diagnostic Arthroscopy

Prior to performing any part of the meniscectomy, it is imperative to always perform a systematic diagnostic arthroscopy of the knee. This practice allows for confirmation of findings noted on physical exam and imaging as well as an opportunity to find any pathology that may have otherwise been missed. The diagnostic arthroscopy should survey seven sections of the knee: medial compartment, lateral compartment, intercondylar notch (cruciate ligaments), patellofemoral articulation, suprapatellar pouch, medial gutter, and lateral gutter. Arthroscopic photographs should be taken of each one of these areas to allow for proper documentation of all damaged tissue. An arthroscopic probe can be utilized in the medial portal to assess the tissues for stability and allow for multiple photographic angles to be taken of found pathology.

With the scope already placed in the medial compartment during its initial introduction into the knee, a valgus force is applied to the leg using the lateral post. This helps to open up the medial compartment and allow for better assessment of the hemijoint. With this valgus force applied, the knee can be flexed or extended appropriately to allow better visualization of various areas within the medial compartment. Once fully assessed, the camera is slowly withdrawn from the medial compartment and driven laterally to assess the notch. The scope is driven into the posterior medial compartment under direct vision. For tighter knees, the posterior medial compartment is more easily entered "blindly" by feel with the blunt obturator. While applying a valgus force and usually moderate flexion, the medial notch is palpated and the obturator is driven into the posterior medial compartment between the medial femoral condyle and the PCL. The presence of peripheral "ramp" type tears may only be appre-

ciated with access through the notch. Once view of the posteromedial compartment is complete, the scope is slowly drawn back in order to visualize the notch. In the notch, the anterior and posterior cruciate ligaments are probed to assess their integrity. After assessing the cruciates, the arthroscope is continued laterally into the lateral hemijoint. In order to open this joint space, a varus stress needs to be applied much in same fashion as a valgus stress helped to open the medial hemijoint. The figure-of-four position is very helpful to achieve this. In addition to the lateral meniscus, the popliteus tendon can be seen in the posterior aspect of the lateral compartment. The popliteal hiatus in this region is a common place to find loose bodies. Similar to medial inspection, the scope may be driven directly into the posterior lateral compartment. For tighter knees, this compartment is best accessed via the contralateral side. Once fully assessed, the camera is again slowly brought back to the region of the intercondylar notch.

This time, the camera is advanced proximally as the knee is carefully extended to allow for visualization of the trochlear groove and patellar undersurface. This proximal direction is terminated in the suprapatellar pouch. Lastly, the camera can be directed over the femoral condyles to assess the medial and lateral gutters with the knee in the fully extended position. This thorough journey through the knee joint allows for a systematic assessment of all aspects of its contents, all via the lateral viewing portal.

Arthroscopic Partial Meniscectomy

After completion of the diagnostic scope, attention should be turned towards performing the partial meniscectomy. First, the tear should be thoroughly assessed with use of the arthroscopic probe.

A principle we attempt to employ is "heavy with the body, easy with the hands." In other words, a leg holder allows considerable leverage with the body to be directed to apply valgus. Using one's body properly allows one to relax and thereby perform optimally. Furthermore, "soft hands" ensure gentleness to tissues. As is taught to the residents, "chondral lesions are forever."

If the tear is displaced (e.g., bucket-handle tear), it should first be reduced with the probe in order to assess its tissue quality as well as facilitating excision—if indicated. Similarly, the probe should be used to pull slight tension on the tear to assess its full extent. This includes probing of the superior and inferior surfaces of the meniscus. Once the tear is defined, the process of excision can proceed.

A useful guideline to optimize the approach to a tear involves the alternating of portals for the arthroscope and instruments. If a tear is located in the posterior aspect of the meniscus, the ipsilateral portal should be used initially for the instruments. Conversely, tears in the anterior aspect of the meniscus should be approached from the contralateral portal. This allows for the instruments to approach the tear at a right angle, or orthogonally, and allow for easier excision.

There are various arthroscopic tools available to the surgeon for excision of the torn meniscus that allows for minimal collateral damage to the remaining normal tissue. The most popular instrument is the arthroscopic suction shaver. Using suction to draw loose tissue into its path, the shaver has an alternating-rotational blade that is suitable for trimming frayed meniscal ridges and excising small tear flaps. The blade of the shaver is usually glided over the area of damaged meniscus in a controlled back and forth motion with slight suction to allow for precise excision. It is important to not leave the shaver running in one region or with excessive suction for too long in order to avoid risk of creating chondral injury. For tighter knees, a curved shaver is often very useful. For larger tear flaps that can displace into the joint, an arthroscopic biter is used to "chew out" the damaged tissue. Biters come in various neck angulations (e.g., straight, right-angled, left-angled) to allow for the most orthogonal approach to the tear. It has been the senior author's experience that smaller upward curves perform better for posterior meniscal lesions, while posterior horn proper is best accessed with the larger upwardly curved biters. Once the larger pieces are freed with the biter, the shaver can then be used to suction up the now free pieces and then to smooth the jagged edges of the recent excision. Alternatively, a thermal ablation device can be used to smooth the edges. The risk of these devices is damage to the articular cartilage, although very smooth resected edges can be attained. Once the excision is completed, the probe should be reinserted into the knee to ensure proper resection of the torn fragment. Final photographs can be taken at this time.

Special Considerations

Horizontal Cleavage Tear

The horizontal cleavage tear is unique in that the upper and lower lamina of meniscal tissue is present. The senior author endeavors to preserve as much stable meniscal tissue as possible. Often most of the lower lamina is sacrificed leaving a nearly intact and stable superior rim. Recent studies suggest that even remaining fragments of meniscal tissue still afford some chondral protection [3].

Radial Tear

Recent data suggest that radial tears left in situ offer more contact stress protection than fully resected tear [4]. Thus, the senior author resects only very unstable elements of radial tears. Repair (see subsequent chapter) is preferred in younger patients.

"Anterior" Lateral Meniscal Tears

Tears of the lateral meniscus that are relatively anterior or involve the anterior horn may be difficult to access. The senior author favors a "look medial/work medial" approach. The most "orthogonal" approach to the anterior horn is via a contralateral accessory medial portal, placed just anterior to the MCL and 5 mm above the joint line. While viewing from a high medial portal, a side biter or shaver from the accessory medial portal will usually suffice. For the most stubborn cases, a "backward biter" introduced from the lateral portal may be necessary.

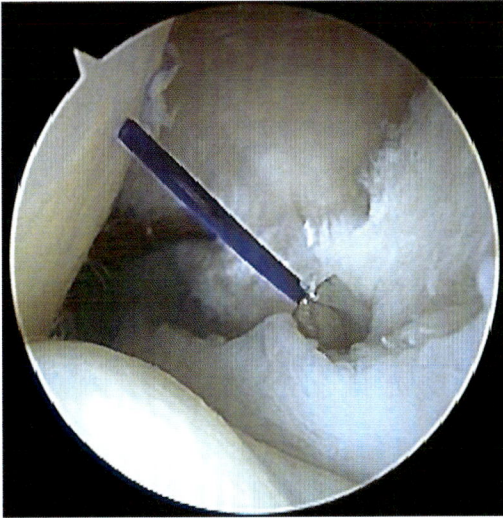

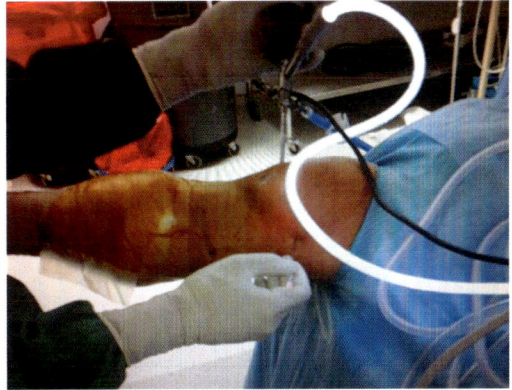

Fig. 4.6 Use of an 18-gauge spinal needle to trephinate the fibers of the MCL under direct arthroscope visualization

Fig. 4.5 Arthroscopic view of the posteromedial compartment of a left knee. A cannulated hook of appropriate curvature loaded with a # 2 PDS resorbable suture thread is introduced into the posteromedial compartment of the knee. The hook is maneuvered so as to purchase the posterior and anterior kissing walls of the entry to the Baker's cyst. After purchasing both cyst walls, the # 2 PDS resorbable suture thread is advanced into the knee joint. The suture of the cyst is performed with the knee bent at 90° so attention should be paid to purchase both walls as caudally as possible in order to prevent the stitches from cutting across soft tissues during extension (Reprinted from Calvisi V. Arthroscopic all-inside suture of symptomatic Baker's cysts: a technical option for surgical treatment in adults. Knee Surg Sport Tr A. 2007 Dec;15(12):1452–60 with permission from Springer)

Baker's Cyst

Rarely a Baker's cyst enlarges to the point of causing posterior knee pain in flexion. If so, the Baker's cyst, which usually accompanies degenerative medial tear and/or medial femoral chondrosis, can be readily excised using one or posterior medial portals [5]. The posterior medial portal is used initially as a working portal so that the cyst origin is "unroofed" between the semimembranosus and the medial gastrocnemius. Once the cyst "valve" is exposed, the scope is driven into the cyst via the anterolateral portal, and a second posterior medial portal is made into the cyst so that the cyst lining may be excised (Fig. 4.5).

Pearls

The "simple meniscectomy" is often not so straightforward. Perhaps the most difficult issue for medial resection is access and visualization. For hard to access medial-sided lesions, the senior author recommends the following algorithmic steps:

1. Release of the MCL with a spinal needle. An 18-gauge spinal needle is used to trephinate the origin of the MCL by using multiple side-to-side piercing motions (Fig. 4.6). If this fails to provide sufficient laxity, a microfracture awl, introduced from a contralateral portal, is used to pierce multiple holes under the medial meniscus and into the deep MCL. Finally, a thermal device may be used ipsilaterally to release the deep MCL and thereby enhance visualization to the superior lamina.

2. Switch to a low medial viewing portal and accessory medial working portal. Viewing from an ipsilateral low medial portal increases access to the posterior horn. An accessory medial working portal, located just anterior to the MCL, will afford excellent working access to the posterior horn.

3. Create a posterior medial portal for instrumentation. In the most stubborn cases, the posterior horn is difficult to access from

the anterior portals. Driving the scope into the posterior compartment via the notch and using a posteromedial portal for a shaver will enable trimming of even the most difficult lesions. The posterior medial portal is placed approximately 2 cm more posterior than usual in order to facilitate access to the posterior horn.

4. Finally, the senior author again emphasizes to consider using a circumferential leg holder as it allows increased leverage and the ability to distract the joint posteriorly. It has truly, in the senior author's opinion, enhanced visualization and reduced the frequency of chondral "scuffs."

Wound Closure and Postoperative Care

The instruments and arthroscope should be removed and the excess fluid massaged out of the portal sites. A non-braided suture (e.g., 3-0 nylon or Prolene) can be used in a figure-of-eight pattern to suture the portal sites closed. Additional intra-articular anesthetic can be given at this time if chosen. The wound is then wrapped in a sterile dressing at the surgeon's preference.

As a stand-alone procedure, arthroscopic partial meniscectomy should not require any significant restrictions on the patient postoperatively. The procedure is typically performed on an outpatient basis and the patient is allowed to weightbear as tolerated immediately with the aid of crutches if needed. There should be no restrictions in range of motion, and a brace is not necessary. If an additional procedure is performed concurrently, such as an ACL reconstruction, then the postoperative restrictions for that procedure take precedence. Pain is typically managed with nonsteroidal anti-inflammatories, limited oral narcotic medications, and cryotherapy as needed. Patients should also begin straight-leg exercises to prevent any quadriceps atrophy. Sutures are typically removed in 7–10 days postoperatively. Patients are typically able to return to full athletic activity within 4–6 weeks.

Outcomes

Arthroscopic partial meniscectomy has shown great success in the literature. Many studies have shown satisfactory clinical results in 80–90 % of patients. Most of these results were based on return of joint function and decrease in pain. In a study by Schimmer et al., 91.8 % of patients reported good or excellent results at 4 years of follow-up. The authors found that the greatest impact on a successful outcome was the observation of articular cartilage damage noted at the time of arthroscopy; only 62 % of patients with noted articular damage reported good to excellent outcomes compared to 94.8 % of patients with no noted articular damage [6]. A 15-year follow-up study by Burks et al. found 88 % good or excellent results in stable knees that underwent arthroscopic partial meniscectomy. In general, results for medial meniscectomy (80–100 % good to excellent) have fared better than those for lateral meniscectomy (54–92 % good to excellent) [2]. Furthermore, some studies suggest a "dose response" of meniscal resection and appearance of later degenerative changes. That is, more meniscal tissue resection usually translates to a higher prevalence of subsequent chondral deterioration. Thus, precise and conservative meniscectomy will serve patients best.

References

1. Miller MD, Cooper DE, Warner JJP, editors. Review of sports medicine and arthroscopy. 2nd ed. Philadelphia, PA: W.B. Saunders; 2002.
2. Burks RT, Metcalf MH, Metcalf RW. Fifteen-year follow-up of arthroscopic partial meniscectomy. Arthroscopy. 1997;13(6):673–9.
3. Bedi A, Kelly NH, Baad M, Fox AJ, Brophy RH, Warren RF, et al. Dynamic contact mechanics of the medial meniscus as a function of radial tear, repair, and partial meniscectomy. J Bone Joint Surg Am. 2010;92(6):1398–408.
4. Vyas D, Harner CD. Meniscus root repair. Sports Med Arthrosc. 2012;20(2):86–94.
5. Takahashi M, Nagano A. Arthroscopic treatment of popliteal cyst and visualization of its cavity through the posterior portal of the knee. Arthroscopy. 2005;21(5):638.
6. Schimmer RC, Brulhart KB, Duff C, Glinz W. Arthroscopic partial meniscectomy: a 12-year follow-up and two-step evaluation of the long-term course. Arthroscopy. 1998;14(2):136–42.

Meniscus Allograft Transplantation

5

Nicole S. Belkin, Brian J. Sennett, and James L. Carey

Abbreviation

MAT   Meniscus allograft transplant or meniscal allograft transplantation

Historical Background

In the early 1900s, the first meniscal allograft procedures were performed in combination with complete knee transplantation, as described by Lexter in 1908 in his work entitled, "Substitute of whole or half-joints from freshly amputated extremities by free plastic operation" [1, 2]. The origins of, or predecessor to, isolated meniscal transplantation can be linked to Gebhardt, who, in 1933, performed fat tissue interposition in an attempt to replace a meniscus

N.S. Belkin, M.D. (✉)
Department of Orthopaedic Surgery, Hospital of the University of Pennsylvania, 3400 Spruce Street, 2 Silverstein, Philadelphia, PA 19104, USA
e-mail: Nicole.Belkin@uphs.upenn.edu

B.J. Sennett, M.D.
Department of Orthopaedic Surgery, Penn Sports Medicine Center, University of Pennsylvania, 235 South 33rd Street, Philadelphia, PA 19104, USA

J.L. Carey, M.D., M.P.H.
Department of Orthopaedic Surgery, Penn Center for Advanced Cartilage Repair and Osteochondritis Dissecans Treatment, Hospital of the University of Pennsylvania, 235 South 33rd Street, Weightman Hall, 1st Floor, Philadelphia, PA 19104, USA

[3]. In more recent history, Locht et al. reported on transplanted parts of the plateau including the meniscus for tibial plateau fractures in 1984 [4]. In the same year, Milachowski had the first reported series of free meniscal allograft transplants in humans [5].

Indications

Meniscus allograft transplantation (MAT) is indicated in a very select subset of patients. Young patients, typically under age 40, who have previously undergone extensive meniscectomy with persistent pain not due to other causes and have failed conservative management, are considered good candidates for MAT. These patients should also have normal mechanical alignment and ligamentous stability of the extremity and relatively normal articular cartilage in the involved compartment, not to exceed Outerbridge I or II changes [6].

Any abnormalities in limb alignment and/or ligamentous stability need to be addressed prior to or concurrently with MAT for successful transplant outcome. Focal cartilage defects can be treated concomitantly, but OAT or ACI procedures should be done following the MAT, to prevent damage to the chondral graft during meniscal implantation [7, 8].

Albeit controversial, some advocates argue that MAT should be considered at time of ACL reconstruction in knees with significant anteromedial rotatory instability from chronic ACL deficiency or failed ACL reconstruction in the presence of deficient medial meniscal tissue, with a goal of providing articular cartilage protection and enhancing joint stability [9]. The posterior horn of the medial meniscus affords appreciable resistance to anterior tibial translation and works synergistically with the ACL in preventing the "pivot shift" phenomenon.

Allograft Sizing

Appropriate sizing of the meniscal graft is an important factor in restoring the biomechanical function of the meniscus. A mismatch in sizing of the allograft has the potential to increase contact pressures and compromise the long-term results of the transplant [10–12].

Therefore, accurate and reproducible sizing methods are essential to the overall success of the meniscal transplant. Currently, the most prevalent methods for sizing meniscal allografts include MRI [13] and radiographic imaging [14]. The utilization of MRI and plain radiographs for determination of graft size has significant deficiencies. These conclusions were confirmed in a study by Shaffer et al. in which the size estimates based on radiographic and MRI images were compared to the actual gross anatomic size of the meniscus, noting significant variability [15]. Improving on the previous methods which focused on measurements derived from imaging modalities, Van Thiel et al. developed and validated a regression model that uses height, weight, and gender variables to accurately predict required allograft meniscal size. This method has been shown to be slightly more accurate in the determination of meniscal size and is the method utilized by our senior author [16]. It is important to note that one should err on the side of oversizing, rather than choose a graft that is marginally small. Slightly larger grafts afford an allowance for the diminution in size or "shrinking" which is known to commonly occur subsequent to transplantation.

Surgical Technique

There are numerous techniques for MAT described in the literature. To allow for a thorough description, we fill focus on describing the senior

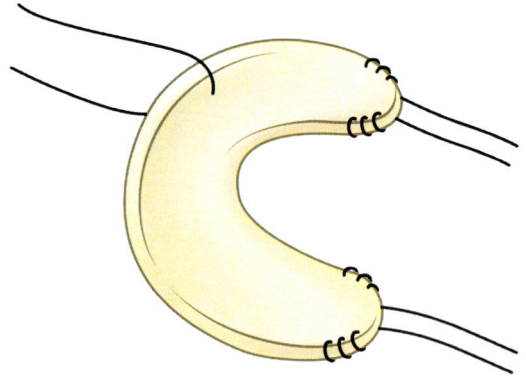

Fig. 5.1 Prepared allograft. A single stitch placed at the junction of the posterior horn and the body and a continuous loop suture is fastened to both horns utilizing a baseball stitch

author's (JBS) preferred technique, which affords direct graft to bone fixation without the need for bone block, and afterward we will briefly discuss alternate methodologies. For a medial meniscal transplantation, the patient is positioned and prepped in the usual fashion for knee arthroscopy with the leg hanging off the side of the table and a lateral post applied. On the back table, the medial meniscus is harvested from the allograft tibial plateau by dissecting the horns free from their boney insertion points. A single stitch with a nonabsorbable braided composite suture (e.g., FiberWire, Arthrex) is placed at the junction of the posterior horn and the body. Then a continuous loop nonabsorbable braided composite suture (e.g., FiberLoop, Arthrex) is fastened to both horns utilizing a baseball stitch (Fig. 5.1). Once the graft is prepared, attention is paid to the recipient site. A standard anterolateral arthroscopic portal is utilized in conjunction with an enlarged, approximately 1 in., anteromedial portal. Utilizing a combination of arthroscopic shaving and biting devices, the residual meniscus is trimmed to a 1 mm width remnant (Fig. 5.2). This remnant serves to enhance the fixation strength achieved at the meniscocapsular junction. The anterior and posterior horn attachment sites on the tibial plateau are identified, and a curette is utilized to debride the superficial bone until bleeding tissue is observed. Then an ACL drill guide is utilized to drill a 2 mm transtibial tunnel from the anterior-medial tibia to the posterior horn attachment site that was just prepared. Suture passing wire (e.g., MicroLasso, Arthrex, Naples, Florida) is placed through this passage into the joint. A helpful hint is to color the tip of the drill guide with ink so that, once removed, the drill hole may be ascertained for Lasso passage. A nitinol wire loop is then introduced into the joint and subsequently retrieved through the tibial tunnel with the suture passing wire. The looped end of the nitinol wire should be out through the enlarged anteromedial portal. Then, the suture that was previously placed in the posterior horn of the allograft is fed through this loop. A meniscal repair needle is passed in an outside-in fashion at the junction of the body and the posterior horn through the meniscal remnant, capsule, soft tissue, and skin. The skin puncture is enlarged with a blade to allow suture passage. Through this needle, a wire with a central eyelet

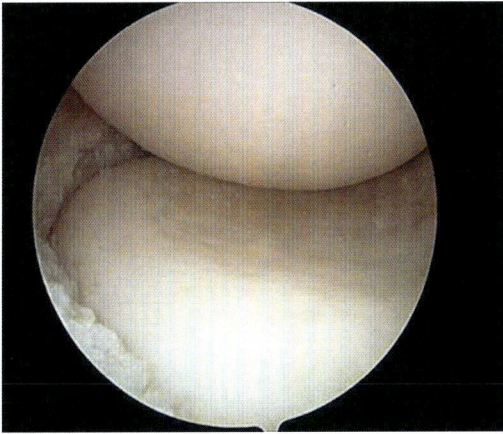

Fig. 5.2 Residual meniscus prepared to accept allograft. Remnant is trimmed to a width of 1 mm

(e.g., Shuttle Relay, ConMed Linvatec) is placed into the joint and then, once the needle is withdrawn, retrieved through the anteromedial portal. This is repeated, resulting in two wires with eyelets passed in through the skin into the joint at the junction of the body and posterior horn of the meniscal remnant and out the anteromedial portal. Each limb of the passing suture that was placed through the allograft initially is placed through an eyelet in one of the wires just placed via the meniscal repair needle. Now the graft can be passed into the joint. The graft is delivered into the joint by pulling on the nitinol wire attached to the posterior horn and then the wires attached to the passing sutures (Fig. 5.3a–c). A lobster or crab claw device should be first passed over both sutures to ensure that no soft tissue bridge exists on the portal. The graft is first fixed at the posterior horn by tying the attached looped suture which has now been passed through the transtibial tunnel over a button on the anteromedial cortex of the tibia. The anterior horn is then fixed utilizing a knotless suture anchor (e.g., PushLock, Arthrex, Naples, Fla.) into the prepared tibial attachment site attached to the looped suture (Fig. 5.4). Access to the anterior horn is best achieved via a high, contralateral lateral portal. Note how both anterior and posterior horns are affixed first before peripheral repair. Then, all-inside meniscal fixation devices (e.g., Fast-Fix, Smith, and Nephew) are utilized to provide fixation within the posterior horn. Vertical mattress sutures, straddling the peripheral rim of the meniscus, render secure fixation. Next, an additional all-inside meniscal fixation device is placed just anterior to the passing sutures.

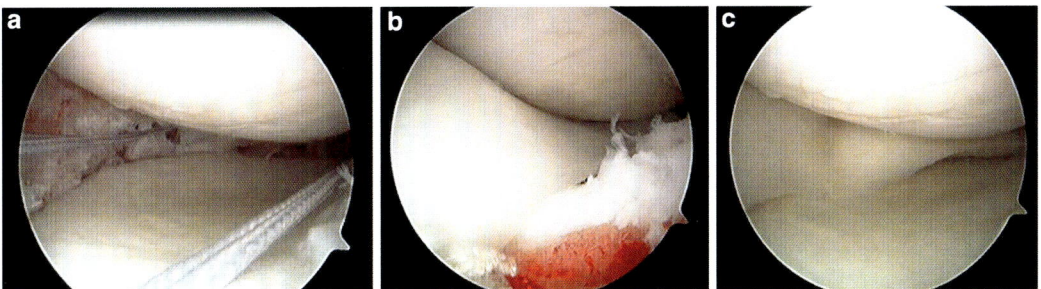

Fig. 5.3 (**a–c**) Delivering the allograft. The graft is pulled into the joint by sequentially pulling on the nitinol wire attached to the posterior horn and then the wires attached to the passing suture

After that, synthetic absorbable monofilament sutures (e.g., 0-PDS, Ethicon) are placed in an outside-in fashion into the anterior horn. Mulberry type knots are fashioned in order to attain meniscal purchase on the inner rim. These sutures are passed through a flap created through the extended medial portal incision. Lastly, an incision is created between the two passing sutures to allow them to be tied under direct visualization, ensuring that the saphenous nerve is not entrapped between them (Fig. 5.5a–b). In cases of incomplete reduction, enlarging the antero-medial portal affords open exposure to the anterior horn whereupon direct suturing, employing double-armed needles, of the anterior horn to the capsule is permitted.

Technical Pearls

1. Exposure is paramount. For medial-sided transplants, MCL release via trephination of the MCL origin, perforation with an awl or thermal release may be necessary. For lateral-sided surgery, a partial "recession" of the popliteus tendon with a thermal device can increase working space greatly.

2. Know your tissue bank. Investigate the "track record" of vendors and compare service and tissue quality.

3. "Back biting" instruments are very useful in removing anterior horn tissue.

4. Ensure that your "suturing" portal for "outside in" or fixators is low enough to permit suture access to the capsular margin. Vertical mattress sutures provide appreciably higher pullout strength than horizontal mattress configuration.

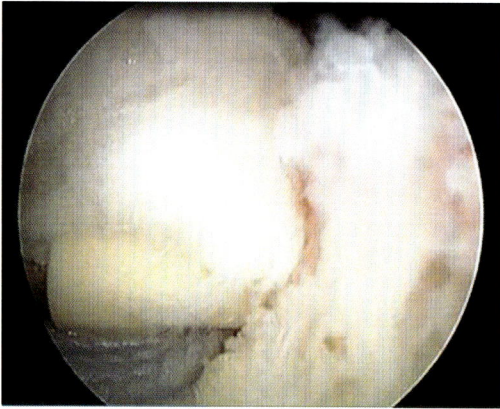

Fig. 5.4 Anterior horn fixation. A continuous loop suture initially placed in the anterior horn is secured to the tibial plateau with a knotless suture anchor

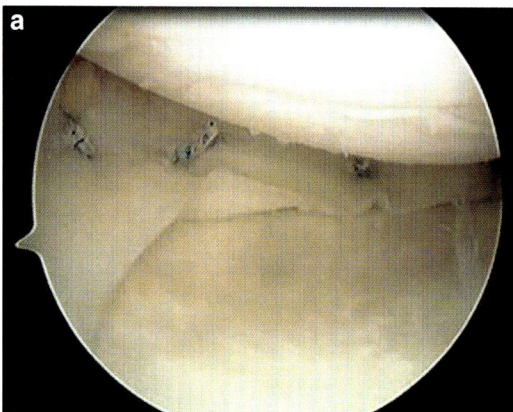

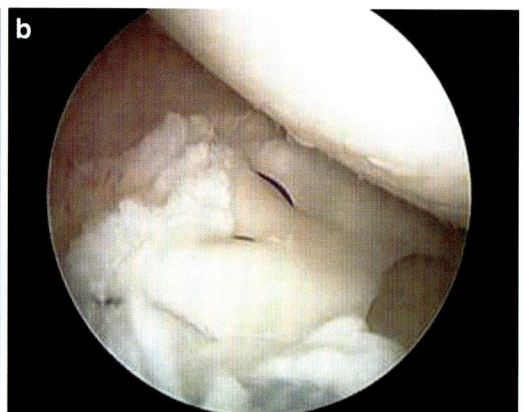

Alternate Techniques

Repeatedly mentioned in the literature is a technique utilizing a dovetail bone block, described as such due to its trapezoidal shape when viewed in the coronal plane. This block, or bridge between

Fig. 5.5 (**a, b**) Peripheral allograft fixation. Two all-inside meniscal fixation devices placed within the posterior horn, then an additional all-inside meniscal fixation device is placed just anterior to the passing sutures, and lastly three synthetic absorbable monofilament sutures are placed in an outside-in fashion into the anterior horn

the anterior and posterior horns, is placed in a congruent slot prepared in the recipient tibia. Also described is a technique utilizing cylindrical bone plugs fashioned at the donor meniscal horn attachments. These plugs are transfixed with suture into tibial tunnels drilled over a guide wire. The senior author has recognized that bone block containing grafts introduce an additional level of difficulty in graft passage. The technique herein described affords direct bone fixation and obviates the need for passage of bulky bone fragments through the joint and subjacent bone tunnels.

For lateral meniscal transplantation, the process is essentially identical, with some differences to consider. The anterior and posterior horn attachments of the lateral meniscus are much more closely approximated than the medial side. Thus, to gain access to the posterior horn of the lateral meniscus, a retractor probe may be necessary to shift the ACL medially in order to visualize the posterior horn drill site. Secondly, since the anterior and posterior horns are in close proximity, one must be mindful not to converge bone tunnels. The authors find that the best angle of approach to the anterior horn is via a high contralateral medial portal.

Although many advocate a "bone bridge" technique for the lateral meniscus transplantation, the authors have not found this necessary and maintain that direct bone fixation is attained in more facile fashion with the above-described technique.

Additional Considerations

As previously discussed, concomitant pathology from injury such as ACL deficiency or chondral defect should be addressed at the time of or prior to meniscal allograft transplantation. Varus and valgus deformity should also be taken into consideration in the setting of meniscal transplantation. In patients with axial malalignment, high tibial osteotomy or distal femoral osteotomy should be performed in conjunction with MAT.

Postoperative Management

For as many operative techniques described, there are twice as many proposed postoperative protocols proposed. At our institution, we prescribe the following restrictions: non-weight bearing for a duration of 6 weeks, to be followed by partial weight bearing with a gradual increase to full weight bearing over the next 2–4 weeks. Discontinuation of crutches is upon resolution of limp. Range of motion is limited to 0–70° for the first 4 weeks, followed by 0–90° for weeks 5 and 6, then increase as tolerated. Aside from aforementioned restrictions, physical therapists are instructed to rehab these patients in the same manner as they do meniscal repair patients. Return to sport is anticipated at 6 month.

Outcomes

The results of meniscal allograft transplantation reported in the literature can be difficult to interpret due to variability in methodology, population heterogeneity, and outcome measures. It should also be noted that the lack of a nonoperative treated control group is considered a fundamental flaw in the reported studies, making it difficult to establish the true chondroprotective effect of this type of treatment.

That being said, a recent systematic review of the literature by Verdonk et al. included 39 studies and sought to investigate the indications, limitations, and results of MAT. In regard to functional outcome following MAT, they reported that all studies showed significant improvement in pain scales and functional activity questionnaires with about 75–90 % of patients experiencing fair to excellent results [17].

Some notable individual studies reported in the literature include Cole et al.'s 2006 2-year follow-up data on 39 patients demonstrating statistically significant improvements in standardized outcome measures and pain and satisfaction scoring and Verdonk et al.'s series of 100 patients in 2005 with 7-year follow-up, reporting an improvement in modified HSS scores from 60.1 to 88.6 [18, 19]. In Chalmer et al.'s retrospective series of 13 high school and higher level athletes with symptomatic meniscal deficiency, they reported a return to desired level of competition in 77 % of their patient's after MAT [20].

Overall, the clinical results of this meniscus allograft transplantation are encouraging and long-lasting in a well-selected patient population who suffered a total meniscectomy. Meniscal allograft appears to becoming the gold standard treatment in this patient population. Although a precise chondroprotective role for MAT has not been clearly elucidated, the fact that clinical scores reflect improvement suggests that, in fact, a disease modification effect may *perhaps* be present.

References

1. Lexer E. Substitute of whole or half-joints from freshly amputated extremities by free plastic operation. Surg Gynecol Obstet. 1908;6:601–7.
2. Wirth CJ. Meniscal transplantation and replacement. In: Fu FH, Harner CD, Vince K, editors. Knee surgery. Baltimore, MD: Lippincott Williams & Wilkins; 1994.
3. von Lewinski G. Basic science. In: Beaufils P, Verdonk R, editors. The meniscus. Springer; 2010.
4. Locht RC, Gross AE, Langer F. Late osteochondral allograft resurfacing for tibial plateau fractures. J Bone Joint Surg Am. 1984;66(3):328–35.
5. Milachowski KA, Weismeier K, Wirth CJ. Homologous meniscus transplantation. Experimental and clinical results. Int Orthop. 1989;13(1):1–11.
6. Erikson E. Editorial. Knee Surg Sports Traumatol Arthrosc. 2006;14(8):694–706.
7. Rodeo SA. Meniscal allografts—where do we stand? Am J Sports Med. 2001;29(2):246–61.
8. Cole BJ, Cohen B. Chondral injuries of the knee. A contemporary view of cartilage restoration. Orthopedics. 2000;6:71–6.
9. Sekiya JK, Giffin JR, Irrgang JJ, Fu FH, Harner CD. Clinical outcomes after combined meniscal allograft transplantation and anterior cruciate ligament reconstruction. Am J Sports Med. 2003;31(6):896–906.
10. Dienst M, Greis PE, Ellis BJ, Bachus KN, Burks RT. Effect of lateral meniscal allograft sizing on contact mechanics of the lateral tibial plateau: an experimental study in human cadaveric knee joints. Am J Sports Med. 2007;35(1):34–42.
11. Haut Donahue TL, Hull ML, Rashid MM, Jacobs CR. The sensitivity of tibiofemoral contact pressure to the size and shape of the lateral and medial menisci. J Orthop Res. 2004;22(4):807–14.
12. Yoon JR, Kim TS, Wang JH, Yun HH, Lim H, Yang JH. Importance of independent measurement of width and length of lateral meniscus during preoperative sizing for meniscal allograft transplantation. Am J Sports Med. 2011;39(7):1541–7.
13. Pollard ME, Kang Q, Berg EE. Radiographic sizing for meniscal transplantation. Arthroscopy. 1995;11(6):684–7.
14. Haut TL, Hull ML, Howell SM. Use of roentgenography and magnetic resonance imaging to predict meniscal geometry determined with a three-dimensional coordinate digitizing system. J Orthop Res. 2000;18(2):228–37.
15. Shaffer B, Kennedy S, Klimkiewicz J, Yao L. Preoperative sizing of meniscal allografts in meniscus transplantation. Am J Sports Med. 2000;28(4):524–33.
16. Van Thiel GS, Verma N, Yanke A, Basu S, Farr J, Cole B. Meniscal allograft size can be predicted by height, weight, and gender. Arthroscopy. 2009;25(7):722–7.
17. Verdonk R, Volpi P, Verdonk P, Van der Bracht H, Van Laer M, Almqvist KF, et al. Indications and limits of meniscal allografts. Injury. 2013;44 Suppl 1:S21–7.
18. Cole BJ, Dennis MG, Lee SJ, Nho SJ, Kalsi RS, Hayden JK, et al. Prospective evaluation of allograft meniscus transplantation: a minimum 2-year follow-up. Am J Sports Med. 2006;34(6):919–27.
19. Verdonk PC, Demurie A, Almqvist KF, Veys EM, Verbruggen G, Verdonk R. Transplantation of viable meniscal allograft. Survivorship analysis and clinical outcome of one hundred cases. J Bone Joint Surg Am. 2005;87(4):715–24.
20. Chalmers PN, Karas V, Sherman SL, Cole BJ. Return to high-level sport after meniscal allograft transplantation. Arthroscopy. 2013;29(3):539–44.

Matthew B. Fisher, Nicole S. Belkin, and Robert L. Mauck

Introduction

Surgery for repair or replacement of the menisci is one of the most common procedures performed in orthopedic surgery, with estimates exceeding one million operations yearly [1, 2]. Suture repair is possible for simple longitudinal tears; however, it is estimated that surgeons only attempt repair in 5–20 % of all treated meniscal injuries [3]. In cases involving complex tears or degeneration, the injured portion of the meniscus is either removed (meniscectomy) or the entire meniscus is replaced using a meniscal allograft [4]. However, meniscectomy does not restore the proper mechanics of the native tissue and can lead to early osteoarthritis (OA) [2, 5, 6]. Even partial meniscectomy has been recently correlated with higher incidence of OA [2, 6].

In cases of failed repair or subtotal meniscectomy, or in cases of persistent pain following meniscectomy, meniscal allograft transplantation is a viable option for young and/or active patients [7]. With appropriate patient selection, the success rates following allograft transplantation vary between 60 and 95 % [8, 9]. While a viable option to alleviate pain and restore function in patients, this procedure suffers from a number of limitations, including availability, potential disease transmission, size matching, and cost as well as the observed decline in tissue properties as remodeling ensues postimplantation [8, 10]. In fact, tissue remodeling may negatively impact the long-term structural viability of such implants. Furthermore, animal studies have yet to provide convincing evidence that meniscal transplantation fully prevents cartilage degradation [11].

In the search for a viable clinical alternative, researchers have developed a variety of scaffolds aimed at replacement of the meniscus. Several of these have gone through clinical trials and have been implemented in clinical practice. Even more scaffolds have been evaluated in in vitro or in preclinical animal models. As previously defined [12], several criteria will be used to assess the success of these scaffolds. First, the scaffold must mimic the complex mechanical properties of the native meniscus as well the native geometry. Second, the scaffolds must be able to positively interact with the biological environment of the knee joint by eliciting a limited immune response, allowing cellular infiltration and matrix production, and integrating with the surrounding tissue. Finally, from a logistical standpoint, the scaffolds must be readily produced, sterilized, and packaged. Additionally, the handling properties must be sufficient so as to allow widespread clinical use without the need for other specialized facilities.

M.B. Fisher, Ph.D. (✉)
Department of Orthopaedic Surgery, University of Pennsylvania, 424 Stemmler Hall, 36th St. & Hamilton Walk, Philadelphia, PA 19104, USA
e-mail: fmatt@mail.med.upenn.edu

N.S. Belkin, M.D.
Department of Orthopaedic Surgery, Hospital of the University of Pennsylvania, 3400 Spruce Street, 2 Silverstein, Philadelphia, PA 19104, USA

R.L. Mauck, Ph.D.
Mckay Orthopaedic Research Laboratory, University of Pennsylvania, Philadelphia, PA, USA

In this chapter, we will discuss these alternative scaffolds in some detail. We will first briefly describe the structure and function of the meniscus, which serves as a guide for any replacement scaffold. This will be followed by a discussion of the types of materials and fabrication techniques available to create scaffolds. Following this primer, we will turn our attention to acellular scaffolds meant to serve as permanent replacements of the meniscus. We will then elaborate on scaffolds in development, with a particular emphasis on the advances in regenerative medicine and tissue engineering. Finally, we will conclude with a discussion of the challenges and future directions for meniscal replacement.

Structure and Function of the Meniscus: A Guide for Replacement Scaffolds

Given the essential role of the menisci in transmitting loads across the knee joint during activities of daily living, the mechanical properties of any replacement scaffold are of paramount importance [13–16]. Due to the unique geometry of the relatively flat tibial plateau and the convex femoral condyles (Fig. 6.1), the wedge-shaped, semilunar menisci are exposed to compression, tension, and shear during normal function [2]. Efforts to develop a replacement scaffold should attempt to match the ability of the native tissue to withstand

these various loading conditions. Typical modulus (measure of stiffness normalized to tissue dimensions) values of the native meniscus in compression and tension are 50–400 kPa and 50–200 MPa, respectively [17–19].

Many replacement scaffolds are designed to degrade overtime and be replaced by host tissue or, if containing a cellular component, to remodel substantially. The long-term success of these scaffolds will be dependent on their ability to induce a new, living tissue with structure similar to the meniscus, which is complex and performs many diverse functions. A brief description of the components of native meniscal tissue will help illustrate the challenges for proper scaffold creation. Meniscus fibrochondrocytes (MFCs) sparsely populate the native tissue and function to maintain and remodel the extracellular matrix (ECM) [20, 21]. Proteoglycans are concentrated in the inner regions where compressive loading predominates [20, 21]. This region also features a mixture of type I and II collagen [20, 21]. Within the outer region, type I collagen predominates to support tensile loading. These collagen fibers are mostly oriented in the circumferential direction (Fig. 6.1), with the occasional radial "tie" fiber or sheet interspersed within this network [22]. The architecture of this collagen component is paramount for meniscus mechanical function. When compressive loads impinge on the wedge-shaped meniscus, an outward tensile load is generated (Fig. 6.1). The circumferential collagen fibers

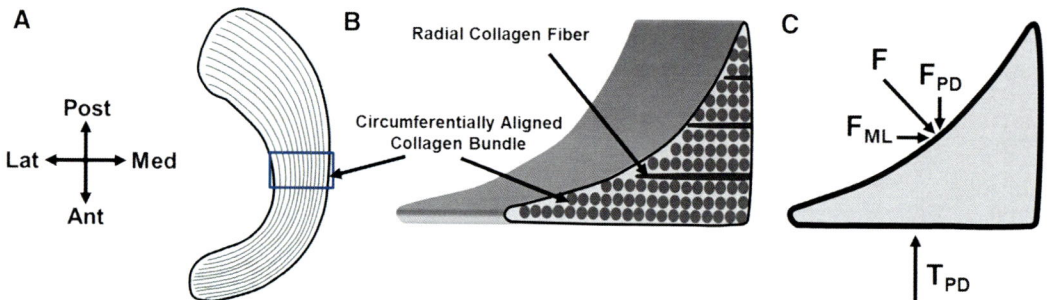

Fig. 6.1 Illustration of meniscus showing generalized anatomic macrostructure (**a**), wedge-like cross section displaying a simplified collagen fiber organization, with the majority of fiber bundles in the circumferential direction with occasional radial "tie" fibers (**b**), and forces acting on the meniscus producing both compressive and tensile loads (**c**) (*F* and *T* correspond to forces from the femur and tibia, respectively. PD and ML represent the proximal-distal and medial-lateral directions, respectively) (Adapted from Fisher et al. [72] with permission from Elsevier)

resist these "hoop stresses" and enforce joint congruency and promote axial load transmission. The success of any "nonpermanent" scaffold will be dependent on its ability to promote new tissue formation with these structural features and hierarchical arrangements.

Types of Materials and Fabrication Techniques

For meniscus replacement scaffolds, two broad classes of materials have been used: synthetic and natural (see Table 6.1 for a list of commonly used materials and fabrication techniques). Synthetic materials consist mainly of polymers, which are biocompatible, easily manufactured, and feature appropriate and modifiable mechanical properties. These include polyvinyl alcohol (PVA), Dacron, polyurethane, polyglycolic acid (PGA), poly-L-lactic acid (PLLA), and polycaprolactone (PCL), among others [23–32].

Alternatively, investigators have created scaffolds made from natural components of the extracellular matrix (ECM). These include tissues directly derived from donors, such as porcine small intestinal submucosa (SIS) [33] or perichondral tissue from the rib [34]. These substances hold the promise of facile incorporation and assimilation. For instance, SIS has shown superiority in cellular interactions versus dermal scaffolds [35]. These submucosal tissues are obtained, decellularized, lyophilized, sterilized, and packaged for direct implantation. One issue is that the decellularization process could result in loss of important biochemical components, such as glycosaminoglycans (GAGs), and as a result, reduced biomechanical properties. As such, a number of "kinder" decellularization techniques are being evaluated [36, 37]. In addition, natural ECM components can be isolated, purified, and utilized as base components for use in similar fabrication methods as synthetic materials. These include type I collagen, glycosaminoglycans, fibrin, and hyaluronic acid [12, 38–41]. As these ECM components naturally interact with cells, the biocompatibility and bioactivity of scaffolds made from such molecules is superior. However, the full complexity of the native ECM environment is likely not achieved. Alternative biological polymers commonly used are agarose, alginate, cellulose, chitosan, and silk [42–46]. Another method is to allow dense cell pellets to make their own matrix, generating a neo-tissue de novo from accumulated matrix molecules [23].

Using these base materials, a number of techniques can be used to form three-dimensional

Table 6.1 Common materials and fabrication techniques used for meniscus scaffolds

	Base material	Fabrication techniques
Synthetic	Poly(ε-caprolactone)	Porous foams [25, 31, 76], nanofibrous assemblies [70]
	Polyvinyl alcohol	Hydrogels [48, 61]
	Polyurethane	Porous foams [25, 27, 31, 62]
	Polyglycolic acid	Nonwoven scaffolds [23, 26, 78]
	Poly-L-lactic acid	Porous foams [29, 32], nonwoven scaffolds [24]
Natural	Collagen (type I, type II, types I/III)	Porous foams [40, 63, 83]
	Hyaluronan/hyaluronic acid	Porous foams [76, 83], hydrogels [39]
	Fibrin	Sealant/hydrogel [74]
	Chondroitin sulfate	Porous foams [40, 41]
	Agarose	Hydrogels [46]
	Alginate	Hydrogels [42, 84]
	Cellulose	Hydrogels [43]
	Chitosan	Self-assembled matrices [41], hydrogels [44]
	Silk	Porous foams [45]
	Small intestinal submucosa	ECM as is (decellularized) [33, 75]
	Perichondral matrix	ECM as is (decellularized) [34]

scaffolds. Foams can be formed by dissolving a polymer into a solution and then placing the solution into a mold and drying it, leaving the remaining polymer. By including a salt solution, pores can be created by placing the scaffolds in an aqueous solution and allowing the salt to be leached from the scaffolds. Alternatively, polymer fibers can be combined together into woven or nonwoven felts with micron-sized fibers using technology borrowed from the textile industry. For scaffolds with fibers on the order of nanometers, a process called electrospinning can be used. Finally, hydrogels are commonly made from a number of materials and feature a large water content, usually >90 %. These gels can be formed into any shape before gelling via changing temperature, pH, electric field, ultrasound, salt concentration, or ultraviolet light. Overall, with the right materials and fabrication methods, compressive properties can be obtained similar to the native tissue [23, 38]. Tensile properties are less widely reported; however, with the proper materials and fabrication methods, mechanical properties approaching that of the native meniscus are possible [47, 48]. Each method has advantages and disadvantages, which have been nicely summarized elsewhere [12, 49]. This chapter will focus on the implementation of the above described materials and fabrication methods to create and evaluate scaffolds for meniscal replacement.

Acellular Permanent Replacements

Early on, several acellular scaffolding materials were evaluated in initial preclinical animal studies, including PLLA foams embedded with carbon fibers [32], Dacron [30], and porous polyurethane [27]. The first alternative meniscal replacement to be used widely is the collagen meniscus implant (CMI), otherwise known as Menaflex® (ReGen Biologics, Inc.). This device is intended as an alternative for partial meniscectomy, especially with the presence of an intact peripheral rim. It was the first device to be approved by the Food & Drug Administration in the USA (although its approval has been rescinded due to an investigation of the initial approval [50]).

This scaffold is produced from a slurry of decellularized bovine Achilles tendon and GAGs, which is molded into a semilunar shape, then lyophilized, chemically cross-linked, and sterilized (Fig. 6.2) [40]. Preclinical data in the dog model suggest the scaffold can allow cellular ingrowth and induce new tissue formation in 63 % of animals at 1 year postoperatively (versus 25 % of no scaffold controls) [40]. Several clinical studies have been published using the CMI device [51–54]. One year after implantation, second-look arthroscopy revealed significant remodeling of the CMI [52]. Through biopsies, clear cellular infiltration and production of a fibrocartilaginous matrix at the edge of the scaffold has been observed. Yet, it is unclear whether this remodeling process occurs throughout the entire CMI.

The most well-known randomized control trial evaluating CMI was performed by Rodkey et al. [52–54]. In over 300 patients, the CMI was directly compared to treatment with a partial medial meniscectomy. Second-look arthroscopy at 1 year postoperatively showed that treatment with the CMI led to significantly more new meniscal tissue compared to partial meniscectomy, and the implant itself was integrated. Interestingly, patients with chronic tears had significantly higher activity levels relative to controls and had lower rates of revision surgeries at an average of 5 years follow-up. However, patients with acute injuries showed no statistically significant impact of the CMI. In addition, there were no reports of chondral wear due to the implant. However, this study has been criticized for certain methodologic flaws. Recently, Monllau et al. have reported long-term outcomes (>10 years) following CMI treatment in a series of 25 patients [51]. Although not controlled, the study showed good or excellent results in 83 % of patients with improved activity and pain levels. However, magnetic resonance imaging revealed shrinking of the implant in 89 % of cases and a failure rate of 8 %.

A more recently developed synthetic scaffold (Actifit; Orteq Bioengineering) is currently on the market in Europe as an alternative for partial meniscectomy. This scaffold, based on a polyurethane/PCL mixture, is lyophilized into a foam-like open pore structure using liquid phase separation

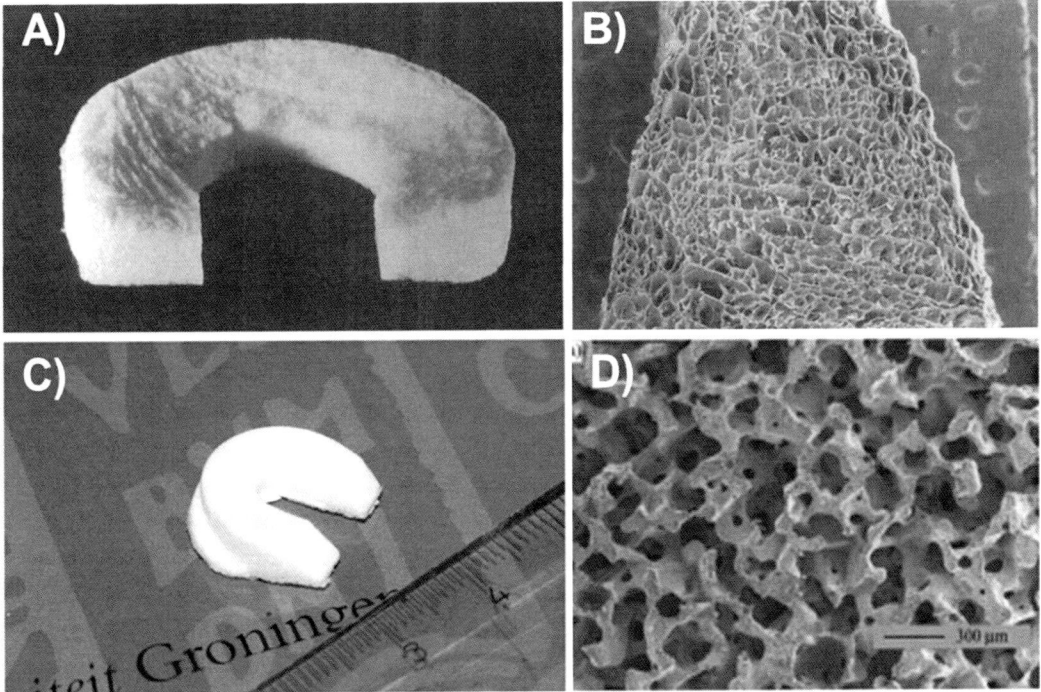

Fig. 6.2 Acellular scaffolds used clinically for meniscus replacement. Collagen meniscus implant (CMI) (**a, b**) and Actifit (**c, d**) scaffolds showing gross appearance (**a, c**) and microstructure (**b, d**) (Adapted from Stone et al. [92] with permission from JBJS and Heijkants et al. [25] with permission from Springer)

and salt leaching techniques, and the final product features a C-shaped geometry and cross-sectional wedge shape (Fig. 6.2) [25, 31]. In a skeletally mature sheep model [55], MRI and histological assessment revealed little to no cartilage damage under the site of scaffold implantation up to 1 year postoperatively. This is supported by in vitro studies in which a similar PCL scaffold could restore contact pressures under the meniscus in the sheep knee joint during a simulated gait movement [14]. Interestingly, however, cartilage damage was found near the midline of the joint in both the Actifit and partial meniscectomy groups, suggesting some altered loading patterns in vivo. These results are mirrored in the dog model of complete meniscus replacement, with cellular infiltration and matrix formation observed at 12 weeks following implantation [25], but a substantial amount of articular cartilage damage found by 6 months [56]. Compressive testing revealed that the behavior of the excised tissue better resembled

the native tissue compared to the original scaffold, although additional improvements are needed to fully replicate the mechanical behavior of the natural structure. Moreover, longer term studies (2 years) showed that the core of the scaffold was acellular, although an ECM remained, bringing the long-term viability of the regenerated tissue into question [57].

The Actifit device was recently evaluated in a case series of more than 50 patients with a previous meniscectomy who still suffered from pain [58]. At 2 years postoperatively, clinical outcome scores (indicating pain, activity levels, and quality of life) were significantly improved relative to preoperative scores. However, failure was noted in 17 % of patients who required reoperation. Biopsy of the scaffold revealed tissue ingrowth and matrix production near the edge of the scaffold [59]. Recent clinical data also highlights the importance of an intact and thick peripheral rim for preventing radial displacement of these scaffolds, particularly when used for replacement of the medial meniscus [60]. With continued use, a controlled study comparing the implant versus meniscectomy is still needed to prove the efficacy of the Actifit scaffold.

Hydrogels made from a PVA hydrogel have also been well studied for meniscus replacement. PVA gels naturally swell in water, leading to high water content (>90 %) and compressive properties similar to the native meniscus. In a rabbit model, implantation of the PVA hydrogel could lessen the degree of cartilage damage up to 2 years compared to meniscectomy, although both groups showed degenerative changes [28]. The PVA hydrogel was able to maintain its mechanical characteristics; however, the ability of this scaffold to integrate with the surrounding tissue was questioned. Kelly et al. used a PVA hydrogel threaded with sutures in a circumferential manner in an ovine model to completely replace the lateral meniscus [61]. Relative to complete meniscectomy, use of the hydrogel led to less cartilage degeneration as assessed via MRI, biomechanical testing, and histology. However, at 4 and 12 months, the hydrogel replacement showed greater cartilage degeneration when compared to a meniscal allograft. In fact, by 12 months, all hydrogels had failed mechanically, with a complete radial fracture in the posterior third of the implant. This study highlights both the need for long-term follow-up in animal models (1 year or more) as well as scaffolds matching both the compressive and tensile properties of the native meniscus. As an initial step toward this goal, Holloway et al. have recently created PVA hydrogels reinforced with ultrahigh molecular weight polyethylene (UHMWPE) fibers to strengthen the tensile mechanics [48]. By modifying the percent composition of the PVA and UHMWPE as well as varying the number of freeze-thaw cycles during fabrication, the scaffolds possessed both compressive and tensile modulus similar to the native meniscus. However, these properties are likely isotropic, i.e., the same in all directions, unlike the native meniscus, which features vastly different properties in the radial and circumferential directions. Similarly,

polycarbonate urethane (PCU) scaffolds reinforced with circumferential Kevlar© (DuPont) fibers have also been used in preliminary studies to replace the entire meniscus in adult sheep ($n = 3$) [62]. Still, long-term large animal studies with a meniscectomy as a control are needed to confirm the effectiveness of these scaffolds.

As a consequence of implant failures, significant efforts have been made in recent years to better match the tensile properties of the meniscus in replacement scaffolds. For example, Balint et al. developed a scaffold comprised of a type I collagen sponge reinforced with resorbable, yet stiff synthetic polymer fibers (poly(desaminotyrosyl-tyrosine dodecyl ester dodecanoate)) [63]. Biomechanical testing in an ex vivo joint model showed that the fiber-reinforced scaffolds could bear compressive loads via the formation of circumferential tensile loads with properties similar to those of the normal ovine meniscus. One limitation of combining materials of varying mechanical characteristics is the possibility of the strong fibers to pull through the potentially fragile hydrogel or foam phase. Another concern is that these large fibers do not mimic the size or number of the collagen fibers in the native meniscus.

One way to instill anisotropic tensile properties uniformly within scaffolds while mimicking the nanofibrous nature of the native ECM is through a process known as electrospinning [64–69]. In particular, electrospun scaffolds made from PCL can match the tensile properties of the native meniscus within the physiological levels of strain [70, 71], and the tensile properties in the aligned direction are more than an order of magnitude higher than in the perpendicular direction. To create scaffolds featuring fibers that are locally aligned but show a continuous change in macroscopic directionality, we recently developed a novel electrospinning method (using a rotating disc mandrel) to produce scaffolds composed of circumferentially aligned (CircAl) nanofibers (Fig. 6.3) [72]. These novel scaffolds, with spatially varying local orientation and mechanics, may enable the formation of functional anatomic meniscus constructs with locally varying fiber architecture to recapitulate native tissue properties.

A   **Linearly Aligned Fibers**

A

B   **Circumferentially Aligned Fibers**

B   SIS   Meniscectomy

C   SIS   Meniscectomy

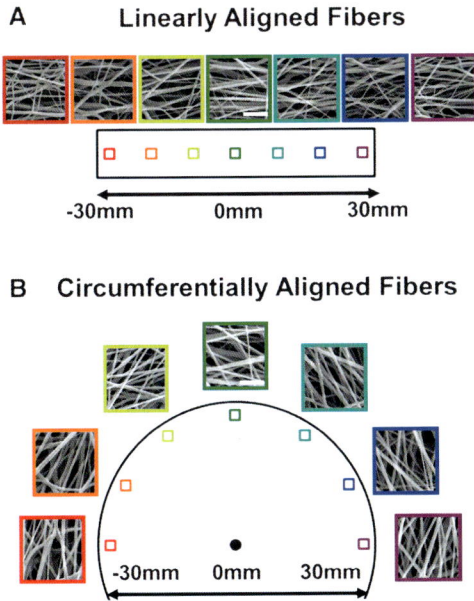

Fig. 6.3 Scanning electron microscopy for linearly aligned (**a**) and circumferentially aligned (**b**) scaffolds (scale bar = 5 μm) (Adapted from Fisher et al. [72] with permission from Elsevier)

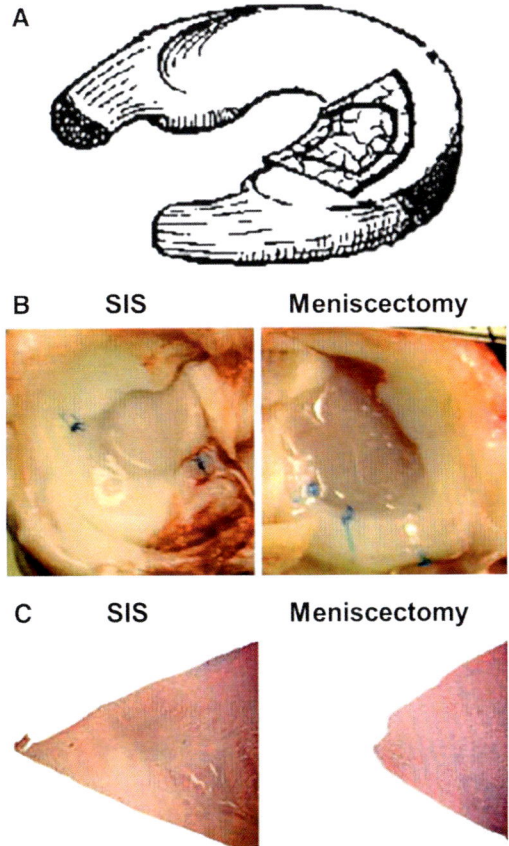

Fig. 6.4 Small intestinal submucosa (SIS) scaffolds for meniscus regeneration. Schematic of scaffold placement (**a**). Gross images (**b**) and histological staining (hematoxylin and eosin) (**c**) of SIS-treated and meniscectomy control menisci at 12 months (Adapted from Cook et al. [33] with permission from SAGE Publications)

Scaffolds for Healing and Regeneration

Instead of designing scaffolds for permanent replacement of the meniscus, some acellular scaffolding materials have been conceived with the purpose of stimulating a healing and regenerative response in vivo. By attracting cells through growth factors and stimulating them to produce new tissue, these scaffolds would be used as a temporary substrate, which would degrade and remodel as the new, and hopefully more permanent, adjunctive tissue forms.

One obvious scaffold is the fibrin clot, which is essential during normal tissue healing in the presence of a blood supply [73]. In pioneering work, Arnoczky et al. created a small full-thickness defect in the avascular portion of the meniscus in the dog model. Interestingly, the fibrin clot was able to support the formation of fibrocartilaginous tissue while untreated defects did not heal. The authors speculate that the reparative cells

originated from the synovial membrane as well as the adjacent meniscal tissue. In later work, Hashimoto et al. added endothelial growth factor to a fibrin sealant and showed increased tissue filling [74]. Despite these positive findings, the histological appearance was still altered relative to normal. Additionally, the ability of a fibrin clot to heal large defects is unlikely.

Other biological scaffolds, such as SIS, have also been used as a graft to promote meniscal regeneration of meniscal defects. Five dogs received grafts and two were left untreated as controls (Fig. 6.4). In a small study in the canine model [75], implantation of the SIS encouraged substantially greater tissue formation at 12 weeks in 80 % dogs with a histological appearance similar to native tissue, including the presence of type II collagen, while untreated control defects filled with fibrous tissue. In a larger follow-up study at 12 months, SIS treatment led to reduced lameness and less secondary cartilage damage [33]. The increase in new tissue formation with SIS observed at 12 weeks was maintained (Fig. 6.4). This tissue was also more mature and better integrated. Still, changes to the articular cartilage were observed in both treatment groups. Additionally, the compressive stiffness of the regenerated tissue, even with SIS treatment, was half that of normal at 1 year follow-up.

Tissue-Engineered Scaffolds

Several research studies have suggested that acellular scaffolds (even ones promoting regeneration) are insufficient to allow incorporation, promote cell infiltration and new matrix production, and improve long-term function [76, 77]. As such, inclusion of cells within scaffolds and culturing in vitro to produce a tissue-like material prior to implantation has been widely pursued and is commonly known as tissue engineering. A number of cell sources are potentially available, including autologous meniscus cells, mesenchymal stem cells (MSCs), xenogeneic cells, embryonic stem cells, and induced pluripotent stem cells. The advantages and disadvantages of each cell type have been detailed elsewhere [12]. To date, no cell type has been approved for treatment of meniscal injuries, but much in vitro and preclinical in vivo work has been carried out to support their use.

In terms of in vivo evaluation, Ibarra et al. performed one of the earliest tissue engineering studies for the meniscus by seeding immature bovine fibrochondrocytes onto nonwoven PGA scaffolds followed by evaluation in the sheep model [26, 78]. More recently, the role of cells pre-seeded onto a scaffold was isolated and explored [76]. In an ovine partial meniscectomy model, the authors compared treatment with a porous hyaluronic acid/PCL scaffold (with PLA

circumferential fibers) alone or seeded with autologous chondrocytes. At 1 year, cellular ingrowth was found from the capsule in all scaffold implants. Histological analysis found cells throughout all constructs (whether originally seeded or not), although a more rounded phenotype was observed in pre-seeded scaffolds (Fig. 6.5). Relative to meniscectomy, the cell-seeded group showed less osteoarthritic changes, although no statistically significant differences could be determined relative to the cell-free scaffold. Martinek et al. investigated the impact of pre-seeding the CMI device with autologous fibrochondrocytes for 3 weeks prior to autologous implantation in the sheep model [77]. After 3 months, the CMI decreased in size with or without cellular pre-seeding. The initial presence of cells also promoted ECM deposition. Interestingly, remodeling was observed in the majority of pre-seeded scaffolds with complete resorption in 25 % of animals. More conclusive in vivo studies are still needed.

Within the laboratory setting, a number of tissue engineering strategies have been investigated. A direct approach is to pack cells in a high density and allow them to produce their own matrix through a "self-assembly" process [79, 80]. Since no additional scaffolds materials are used, the resulting construct consists entirely of the cells and the natural ECM they produce. Co-cultures of meniscal fibrochondrocytes (MFCs) and articular chondrocytes (ACs) seeded into ring-shaped agarose wells produced matrix resulting in a 4× higher tensile modulus in the circumferential direction relative to the radial direction by 8 weeks [23]. Further benefits of treatment with anabolic and catabolic agents [80] as well as mechanical stimulation of these scaffolds have been shown [81]. However, the tensile properties of the produced tissue are still several orders of magnitude lower than the native meniscus.

ECM-based scaffolds have also been combined with cells for meniscus tissue engineering applications. Mueller et al. seeded bovine meniscus cells within scaffolds made of GAGs and type I or type II collagen. Interestingly, the presence of type II collagen encouraged cell proliferation, increased GAG synthesis, and thwarted

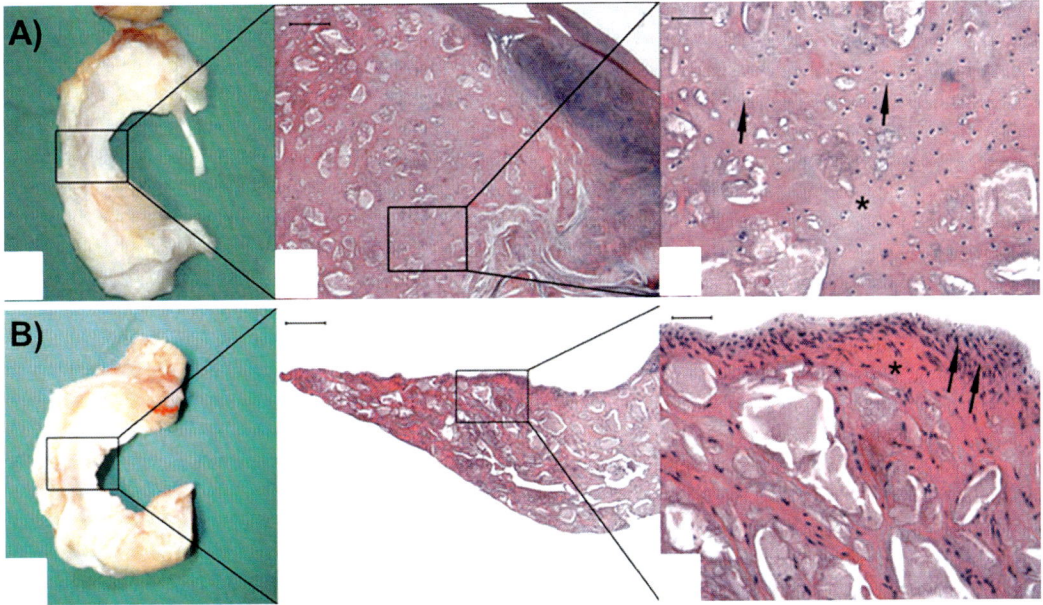

Fig. 6.5 Example of a tissue-engineered scaffold for meniscus replacement in vivo. Images of a cell-seeded implant (**a**) and cell-free implant (**b**) at 12 months postoperatively, including a macroscopic image and histological staining (hematoxylin and eosin) (scale bars = 500 and 100 μm for low and high magnification images, respectively) (Adapted with permission from Kon et al. [76]: the publisher for this copyrighted material is Mary Ann Liebert, Inc. Publishers)

tissue contraction relative to scaffolds containing type I collagen over a 3 week course [82]. In a similar study, Chiari et al. seeded ovine meniscal cells on biomaterials made from a bilayer collagenous scaffold (type II/type I, III) or hyaluronan (Hyaff-11) [83]. Both scaffold types supported cell adhesion and proliferation as well as meniscus-specific matrix production, including GAG and collagen type I. However, the authors found little collagen type II production. More complex scaffolds composed of a hyaluronic acid, chitosan, collagen types I and II, and chondroitin-6-sulfate have also been used in short-term in vitro studies with rat meniscal fibrochondrocytes [41].

Cell-seeded hydrogels have also been utilized as a meniscus replacement scaffold. Some have used computed tomography or MRI to create molds that mimic the geometry of the meniscus and serve as a template from which hydrogels with unique geometry can be formed [38, 84]. Using such a system, Ballyns et al. suspended bovine meniscal fibrochondrocytes within an alginate hydrogel shaped like the sheep meniscus [42, 84]. A custom bioreactor was also designed to provide dynamic compression and further improve these properties [38]. With 2 weeks of dynamic loading, two- to threefold increases in ECM content and compressive modulus were observed. However, by 6 weeks, both GAG content and compressive modulus decreased relative to 2 weeks, suggesting that long-term loading likely had a negative effect. The tensile properties of these constructs still remain orders of magnitude lower than the native tissue. Alternatively, others have utilized silk-based scaffolds for meniscus tissue engineering, partly due to the high tensile strength of silk. Mandal et al. fabricated a multilayered wedge-shaped silk scaffold featuring individual layers with different pore sizes and orientations [45]. These scaffolds supported the formation of matrix containing GAGs and collagen types I and II.

Our lab has utilized scaffolds manufactured by an electrospin nanofiber production technique to produce tissue-engineered meniscus constructs

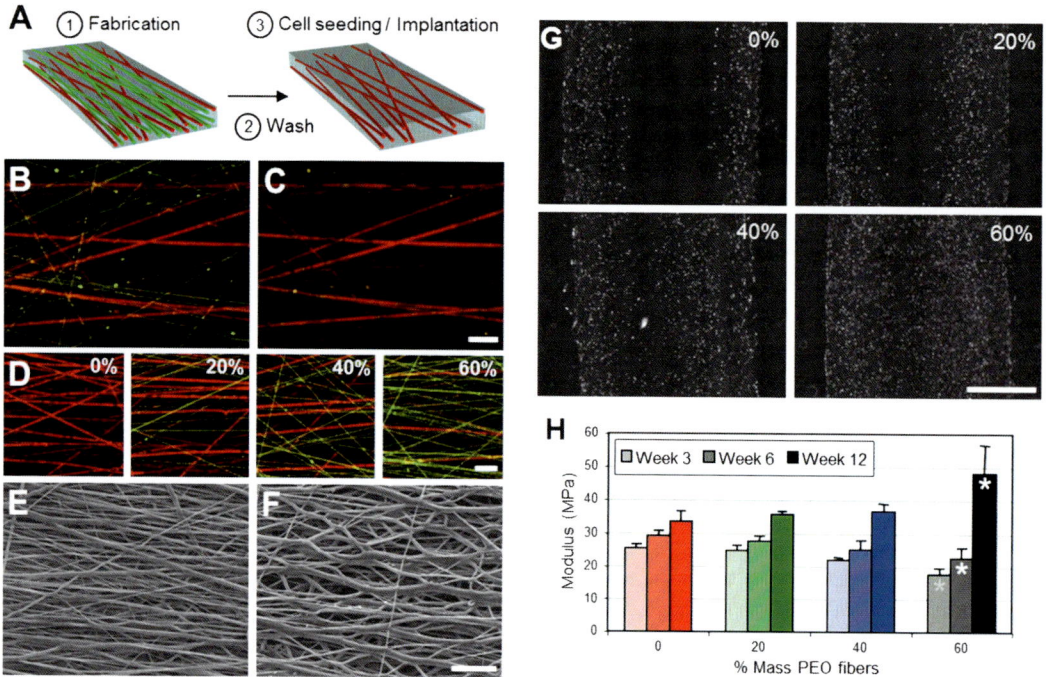

Fig. 6.6 Aligned composite nanofibrous scaffolds for meniscus tissue engineering. Schematic depicting scaffold fabrication and subsequent removal of a sacrificial fiber subpopulation (**a**). Slow-eroding PCL (*red*) and water-soluble PEO (*green*) fibers in composite scaffolds (**b**). In a humid environment, PEO fibers began to dissolve (**c**). Composites with a range of sacrificial fiber inclusion (% indicates PEO content) (**d**). SEM images of scaffolds containing low (0 %) (**e**) and high (60 %) (**f**) sacrificial fiber fractions after hydration (scale bars: 10 μm).

Removal of sacrificial fibers promotes cell infiltration in nanofibrous composites (**g**). Cross sections from constructs containing 0, 20, 40, and 60 % PEO (by mass) showing cell nuclei (scale bar: 500 μm). Long-term culture of composite nanofibrous scaffolds with high sacrificial content results in improved mechanical function (modulus) (**h**) (*$P < 0.05$ compared with time point-matched 0 % constructs) (Adapted with permission from Baker et al. [47] and the National Academy of Sciences of the United States of America)

seeded with cells. In one recent study, we found that nanofiber-aligned scaffolds seeded with either MSCs or MFCs saw almost a 100 % increase in tensile properties over 10 weeks of culture, while unaligned constructs increased by only 20 % [70]. On aligned scaffolds, polarized light microscopy showed ordered collagen deposition, whereas deposited collagen was disorganized on nonaligned scaffolds. Follow-up studies have shown similar effects using human meniscus cells [85]. As a method to increase pore sizes in electrospun scaffolds, we recently fabricated dual-polymer constructs with two polymers, PCL as above, and PEO, which rapidly dissolves in an aqueous environment (Fig. 6.6) [47, 86]. Over 12 weeks, significantly higher fractions of human MFCs were able to migrate into the more

central regions of the scaffolds with increased PEO content. Most interestingly, the ability to allow cellular infiltration resulted in larger increases in construct mechanics over the culture period, reaching levels on the order of the native meniscus. This increased porosity also improved integration with the native meniscus in an in vitro explant model [87, 88]. Ongoing studies are evaluating how these scaffolds operate within the challenging environment within the knee.

Conclusion and Future Focus

An understanding of the important role of the meniscus has come a long way from the initial pioneering work by Fairbank in the mid-1900s [89].

It is now accepted that even partial removal of the meniscus leads to an increased risk of osteoarthritis [90]. Despite this knowledge, meniscectomy is still the most commonly performed orthopedic surgical procedure. In order to improve outcomes in the case of complex injuries not amenable to suture repair, a number of scaffolds have been developed to replace large portions or the entire meniscus. These have been constructed from a variety of synthetic and natural materials with the goal of either structurally replacing the meniscus entirely or promoting the generation of new tissue. Additionally, tissue engineering techniques afford the ability for cells to become isolated and added to these scaffolds and subsequently cultured in vitro to create living tissue analogs prior to implantation.

The progress to date underscores the importance of an appropriate scaffold material. Two acellular scaffolds (CMI and Actifit) have been used clinically as an alternative to partial meniscectomy with encouraging clinical findings [58, 91], yet challenges remain. In 2008, the CMI became the first product available in the USA before its approval was revoked in 2010 by the FDA [50]. Since then, no meniscal replacement scaffolds have been approved by the FDA. Future success of any scaffold for meniscus replacement/augmentation will depend on the efforts of several parties, including industry, regulatory bodies, clinicians, and patients.

Despite these hurdles, there is considerable reason for hope that new scaffolds could have a profound impact on clinical treatment of meniscal injuries. Increasingly sophisticated scaffolds are being developed to match the complex mechanical properties of the meniscus as well as promote a superior biological response to enhance long-term function. One exciting development is the release of growth factors from scaffolds in a spatiotemporal manner to recruit cells, promote infiltration, and direct appropriate matrix production. Further enhancement of tissue incorporation can be realized by working to control degradation of the scaffolds during the healing process. Inclusion of multiple cell types within a single scaffold can also mimic the regional variation in cell phenotype observed in the native meniscus. In the future, it will be critical to perform comprehensive in vivo studies to validate the exciting in vitro progress to date. Vital remaining questions include the following: "is it better to regenerate the meniscus in vivo or develop a meniscus-like tissue in vitro?" "What is the best cell type to include within these scaffolds?" "When is the optimal time for implantation in terms of construct maturity?" "Should mechanical loading be applied following implantation, and if so, how much?" Ultimately, controlled clinical studies will provide the definitive proof of the effectiveness of these approaches. These are exciting times as a multitude of promising scaffold alternatives are on the verge of being available to enhance outcomes after injury to the meniscus.

Acknowledgements We gratefully acknowledge support from the National Institutes of Health (R01EB02425, R01AR056624), the Veterans' Administration (I01RX000174), Musculoskeletal Transplant Foundation (Junior Investigator Grant), the Orthopaedic Research and Education Foundation, the Penn Center for Musculoskeletal Disorders (P30AR050950), and the Penn Institute for Regenerative Medicine.

References

1. Greis PE, Holmstrom MC, Bardana DD, Burks RT. Meniscal injury: II. Management. J Am Acad Orthop Surg. 2002;10(3):177–87.
2. Rath E, Richmond JC. The menisci: basic science and advances in treatment. Br J Sports Med. 2000;34(4):252–7.
3. DeHaven KE. Meniscus repair. Am J Sports Med. 1999;27(2):242–50.
4. Jackson DW, Simon TM. Biology of meniscal allograft. In: Mow VC, Arnoczky SP, Jackson DW, editors. Knee meniscus: basic and clinical foundations. New York: Raven; 1992. p. 141–52.
5. Ahmed AM. The load-bearing role of the knee meniscus. In: Mow VC, Arnoczky SP, Jackson DW, editors. Knee meniscus: basic and clinical foundations. New York: Raven; 1992. p. 59–73.
6. Petrosini AV, Sherman OH. A historical perspective on meniscal repair. Clin Sports Med. 1996;15(3):445–53.
7. Cole BJ, Carter TR, Rodeo SA. Allograft meniscal transplantation: background, techniques, and results. Instr Course Lect. 2003;52:383–96.
8. Elattar M, Dhollander A, Verdonk R, Almqvist KF, Verdonk P. Twenty-six years of meniscal allograft

transplantation: is it still experimental? A meta-analysis of 44 trials. Knee Surg Sports Traumatol Arthrosc. 2011;19(2):147–57.

9. Packer JD, Rodeo SA. Meniscal allograft transplantation. Clin Sports Med. 2009;28(2):259–83. viii.

10. Verdonk P, Depaepe Y, Desmyter S, De Muynck M, Almqvist KF, Verstraete K, et al. Normal and transplanted lateral knee menisci: evaluation of extrusion using magnetic resonance imaging and ultrasound. Knee Surg Sports Traumatol Arthrosc. 2004;12(5): 411–9.

11. Kelly BT, Potter HG, Deng XH, Pearle AD, Turner AS, Warren RF, et al. Meniscal allograft transplantation in the sheep knee: evaluation of chondroprotective effects. Am J Sports Med. 2006;34(9):1464–77.

12. Makris EA, Hadidi P, Athanasiou KA. The knee meniscus: structure-function, pathophysiology, current repair techniques, and prospects for regeneration. Biomaterials. 2011;32(30):7411–31.

13. Ahmed AM, Burke DL. In-vitro measurement of static pressure distribution in synovial joints—Part I: Tibial surface of the knee. J Biomech Eng. 1983; 105(3):216–25.

14. Bedi A, Kelly NH, Baad M, Fox AJ, Brophy RH, Warren RF, et al. Dynamic contact mechanics of the medial meniscus as a function of radial tear, repair, and partial meniscectomy. J Bone Joint Surg Am. 2010;92(6):1398–408.

15. Fukubayashi T, Kurosawa H. The contact area and pressure distribution pattern of the knee. A study of normal and osteoarthrotic knee joints. Acta Orthop Scand. 1980;51(6):871–9.

16. Hunter SA, Rapoport HS, Connolly JM, Alferiev I, Fulmer J, Murti BH, et al. Biomechanical and biologic effects of meniscus stabilization using triglycidyl amine. J Biomed Mater Res A. 2010;93(1): 235–42.

17. Bursac P, Arnoczky S, York A. Dynamic compressive behavior of human meniscus correlates with its extracellular matrix composition. Biorheology. 2009;46(3): 227–37.

18. Bursac P, York A, Kuznia P, Brown LM, Arnoczky SP. Influence of donor age on the biomechanical and biochemical properties of human meniscal allografts. Am J Sports Med. 2009;37(5):884–9.

19. Proctor CS, Schmidt MB, Whipple RR, Kelly MA, Mow VC. Material properties of the normal medial bovine meniscus. J Orthop Res. 1989;7(6):771–82.

20. Adams ME, Hukins DWL. The extracellular matrix of the meniscus. In: Mow VC, Arnoczky SP, Jackson DW, editors. Knee meniscus: basic and clinical foundations. New York: Raven; 1992. p. 15–28.

21. McDevitt CA, Webber RJ. The ultrastructure and biochemistry of meniscal cartilage. Clin Orthop Relat Res. 1990;252:8–18.

22. Petersen W, Tillmann B. Collagenous fibril texture of the human knee joint menisci. Anat Embryol (Berl). 1998;197(4):317–24.

23. Aufderheide AC, Athanasiou KA. Assessment of a bovine co-culture, scaffold-free method for growing meniscus-shaped constructs. Tissue Eng. 2007;13(9): 2195–205.

24. Gunja NJ, Uthamanthil RK, Athanasiou KA. Effects of TGF-beta1 and hydrostatic pressure on meniscus cell-seeded scaffolds. Biomaterials. 2009;30(4): 565–73.

25. Heijkants RG, van Calck RV, De Groot JH, Pennings AJ, Schouten AJ, van Tienen TG, et al. Design, synthesis and properties of a degradable polyurethane scaffold for meniscus regeneration. J Mater Sci Mater Med. 2004;15(4):423–7.

26. Ibarra C, Koski JA, Warren RF. Tissue engineering meniscus: cells and matrix. Orthop Clin North Am. 2000;31(3):411–8.

27. Klompmaker J, Veth RP, Jansen HW, Nielsen HK, de Groot JH, Pennings AJ, et al. Meniscal repair by fibrocartilage in the dog: characterization of the repair tissue and the role of vascularity. Biomaterials. 1996;17(17):1685–91.

28. Kobayashi M, Chang YS, Oka M. A two year in vivo study of polyvinyl alcohol-hydrogel (PVA-H) artificial meniscus. Biomaterials. 2005;26(16):3243–8.

29. Silva MM, Cyster LA, Barry JJ, Yang XB, Oreffo RO, Grant DM, et al. The effect of anisotropic architecture on cell and tissue infiltration into tissue engineering scaffolds. Biomaterials. 2006;27(35):5909–17.

30. Sommerlath KG, Gillquist J. The effect of anterior cruciate ligament resection and immediate or delayed implantation of a meniscus prosthesis on knee joint biomechanics and cartilage. An experimental study in rabbits. Clin Orthop Relat Res. 1993;289:267–75.

31. van Tienen TG, Heijkants RG, Buma P, de Groot JH, Pennings AJ, Veth RP. Tissue ingrowth and degradation of two biodegradable porous polymers with different porosities and pore sizes. Biomaterials. 2002;23(8):1731–8.

32. Veth RP, Jansen HW, Leenslag JW, Pennings AJ, Hartel RM, Nielsen HK. Experimental meniscal lesions reconstructed with a carbon fiber-polyurethane-poly(L-lactide) graft. Clin Orthop Relat Res. 1986;202:286–93.

33. Cook JL, Fox DB, Malaviya P, Tomlinson JL, Kuroki K, Cook CR, et al. Long-term outcome for large meniscal defects treated with small intestinal submucosa in a dog model. Am J Sports Med. 2006;34(1): 32–42.

34. Bruns J, Kahrs J, Kampen J, Behrens P, Plitz W. Autologous perichondral tissue for meniscal replacement. J Bone Joint Surg Br. 1998;80(5):918–23.

35. Cook JL, Fox DB, Kuroki K, Jayo M, De Deyne PG. In vitro and in vivo comparison of five biomaterials used for orthopedic soft tissue augmentation. Am J Vet Res. 2008;69(1):148–56.

36. Crapo PM, Gilbert TW, Badylak SF. An overview of tissue and whole organ decellularization processes. Biomaterials. 2011;32(12):3233–43.

37. Sandmann GH, Eichhorn S, Vogt S, Adamczyk C, Aryee S, Hoberg M, et al. Generation and characterization of a human acellular meniscus scaffold for

tissue engineering. J Biomed Mater Res A. 2009; 91(2):567–74.

38. Ballyns JJ, Bonassar LJ. Dynamic compressive loading of image-guided tissue engineered meniscal constructs. J Biomech. 2011;44(3):509–16.

39. Chen JP, Cheng TH. Preparation and evaluation of thermo-reversible copolymer hydrogels containing chitosan and hyaluronic acid as injectable cell carriers. Polymer. 2009;50(1):107–16.

40. Stone KR, Rodkey WG, Webber R, McKinney L, Steadman JR. Meniscal regeneration with copolymeric collagen scaffolds. In vitro and in vivo studies evaluated clinically, histologically, and biochemically. Am J Sports Med. 1992;20(2):104–11.

41. Tan GK, Dinnes DL, Butler LN, Cooper-White JJ. Interactions between meniscal cells and a self assembled biomimetic surface composed of hyaluronic acid, chitosan and meniscal extracellular matrix molecules. Biomaterials. 2010;31(23): 6104–18.

42. Ballyns JJ, Wright TM, Bonassar LJ. Effect of media mixing on ECM assembly and mechanical properties of anatomically-shaped tissue engineered meniscus. Biomaterials. 2011;31(26):6756–63.

43. Bodin A, Concaro S, Brittberg M, Gatenholm P. Bacterial cellulose as a potential meniscus implant. J Tissue Eng Regen Med. 2007;1(5):406–8.

44. Chen JP, Cheng TH. Thermo-responsive chitosan-graft-poly(N-isopropylacrylamide) injectable hydrogel for cultivation of chondrocytes and meniscus cells. Macromol Biosci. 2006;6(12):1026–39.

45. Mandal BB, Park SH, Gil ES, Kaplan DL. Multilayered silk scaffolds for meniscus tissue engineering. Biomaterials. 2012;32(2):639–51.

46. Wilson CG, Nishimuta JF, Levenston ME. Chondrocytes and meniscal fibrochondrocytes differentially process aggrecan during de novo extracellular matrix assembly. Tissue Eng Part A. 2009;15(7): 1513–22.

47. Baker BM, Shah RP, Silverstein AM, Esterhai JL, Burdick JA, Mauck RL. Sacrificial nanofibrous composites provide instruction without impediment and enable functional tissue formation. Proc Natl Acad Sci U S A. 2012;109(35):14176–81.

48. Holloway JL, Lowman AM, Palmese GR. Mechanical evaluation of poly(vinyl alcohol)-based fibrous composites as biomaterials for meniscal tissue replacement. Acta Biomater. 2010;6(12):4716–24.

49. Baker BM, Gee AO, Sheth NP, Huffman GR, Sennett BJ, Schaer TP, et al. Meniscus tissue engineering on the nanoscale: from basic principles to clinical application. J Knee Surg. 2009;22(1):45–59.

50. FDA. FDA determines knee device should not have been cleared for marketing [Internet]. 2010 [updated 2013 Apr 19]. Available from: http://www.fda.gov/NewsEvents/Newsroom/PressAnnouncements/2010/ucm229384.htm.

51. Monllau JC, Gelber PE, Abat F, Pelfort X, Abad R, Hinarejos P, et al. Outcome after partial medial meniscus substitution with the collagen meniscal implant at a minimum of 10 years' follow-up. Arthroscopy. 2011;27(7):933–43.

52. Rodkey WG, Steadman JR, Li ST. A clinical study of collagen meniscus implants to restore the injured meniscus. Clin Orthop Relat Res 1999;367 Suppl:S281–92.

53. Rodkey WG, DeHaven KE, Montgomery III WH, Baker Jr CL, Beck Jr CL, Hormel SE, et al. Comparison of the collagen meniscus implant with partial meniscectomy. A prospective randomized trial. J Bone Joint Surg Am. 2008;90(7):1413–26.

54. Steadman JR, Rodkey WG. Tissue-engineered collagen meniscus implants: 5- to 6-year feasibility study results. Arthroscopy. 2005;21(5):515–25.

55. Maher SA, Rodeo SA, Doty SB, Brophy R, Potter H, Foo LF, et al. Evaluation of a porous polyurethane scaffold in a partial meniscal defect ovine model. Arthroscopy. 2010;26(11):1510–9.

56. Tienen TG, Heijkants RG, de Groot JH, Pennings AJ, Schouten AJ, Veth RP, et al. Replacement of the knee meniscus by a porous polymer implant: a study in dogs. Am J Sports Med. 2006;34(1):64–71.

57. Welsing RT, van Tienen TG, Ramrattan N, Heijkants R, Schouten AJ, Veth RP, et al. Effect on tissue differentiation and articular cartilage degradation of a polymer meniscus implant: a 2-year follow-up study in dogs. Am J Sports Med. 2008;36(10):1978–89.

58. Verdonk P, Beaufils P, Bellemans J, Djian P, Heinrichs EL, Huysse W, et al. Successful treatment of painful irreparable partial meniscal defects with a polyurethane scaffold: two-year safety and clinical outcomes. Am J Sports Med. 2012;40(4):844–53.

59. Verdonk R, Verdonk P, Huysse W, Forsyth R, Heinrichs EL. Tissue ingrowth after implantation of a novel, biodegradable polyurethane scaffold for treatment of partial meniscal lesions. Am J Sports Med. 2011;39(4):774–82.

60. De Coninck T, Huysse W, Willemot L, Verdonk R, Verstraete K, Verdonk P. Two-year follow-up study on clinical and radiological outcomes of polyurethane meniscal scaffolds. Am J Sports Med. 2013;41(1): 64–72.

61. Kelly BT, Robertson W, Potter HG, Deng XH, Turner AS, Lyman S, et al. Hydrogel meniscal replacement in the sheep knee: preliminary evaluation of chondroprotective effects. Am J Sports Med. 2007; 35(1):43–52.

62. Zur G, Linder-Ganz E, Elsner JJ, Shani J, Brenner O, Agar G, et al. Chondroprotective effects of a polycarbonate-urethane meniscal implant: histopathological results in a sheep model. Knee Surg Sports Traumatol Arthrosc. 2011;19(2):255–63.

63. Balint E, Gatt Jr CJ, Dunn MG. Design and mechanical evaluation of a novel fiber-reinforced scaffold for meniscus replacement. J Biomed Mater Res A. 2012;100(1):195–202.

64. Barnes CP, Sell SA, Boland ED, Simpson DG, Bowlin GL. Nanofiber technology: designing the next generation of tissue engineering scaffolds. Adv Drug Deliv Rev. 2007;59(14):1413–33.

65. Li D, Xia YN. Electrospinning of nanofibers: reinventing the wheel? Adv Mater. 2004;16(14):1151–70.

66. Li WJ, Mauck RL, Tuan RS. Electrospun nanofibrous scaffolds: production, characterization, and applications for tissue engineering and drug delivery. J Biomed Nanotechnol. 2005;1(3):259–75.

67. Mauck RL, Baker BM, Nerurkar NL, Burdick JA, Li WJ, Tuan RS, et al. Engineering on the straight and narrow: the mechanics of nanofibrous assemblies for fiber-reinforced tissue regeneration. Tissue Eng Part B Rev. 2009;15(2):171–93.

68. Pham QP, Sharma U, Mikos AG. Electrospinning of polymeric nanofibers for tissue engineering applications: a review. Tissue Eng. 2006;12(5):1197–211.

69. Stella JA, D'Amore A, Wagner WR, Sacks MS. On the biomechanical function of scaffolds for engineering load-bearing soft tissues. Acta Biomater. 2010;6(7):2365–81.

70. Baker BM, Mauck RL. The effect of nanofiber alignment on the maturation of engineered meniscus constructs. Biomaterials. 2007;28(11):1967–77.

71. Li WJ, Mauck RL, Cooper JA, Yuan X, Tuan RS. Engineering controllable anisotropy in electrospun biodegradable nanofibrous scaffolds for musculoskeletal tissue engineering. J Biomech. 2007;40(8):1686–93.

72. Fisher MB, Henning EA, Soegaard N, Esterhai JL, Mauck RL. Organized nanofibrous scaffolds that mimic the macroscopic and microscopic architecture of the knee meniscus. Acta Biomater. 2013;9(1):4496–504.

73. Arnoczky SP, Warren RF, Spivak JM. Meniscal repair using an exogenous fibrin clot. An experimental study in dogs. J Bone Joint Surg Am. 1988;70(8):1209–17.

74. Hashimoto J, Kurosaka M, Yoshiya S, Hirohata K. Meniscal repair using fibrin sealant and endothelial cell growth factor. An experimental study in dogs. Am J Sports Med. 1992;20(5):537–41.

75. Cook JL, Tomlinson JL, Kreeger JM, Cook CR. Induction of meniscal regeneration in dogs using a novel biomaterial. Am J Sports Med. 1999;27(5):658–65.

76. Kon E, Filardo G, Tschon M, Fini M, Giavaresi G, Marchesini Reggiani L, et al. Tissue engineering for total meniscal substitution: animal study in sheep model—results at 12 months. Tissue Eng Part A. 2012;18(15–16):1573–82.

77. Martinek V, Ueblacker P, Braun K, Nitschke S, Mannhardt R, Specht K, et al. Second generation of meniscus transplantation: in-vivo study with tissue engineered meniscus replacement. Arch Orthop Trauma Surg. 2006;126(4):228–34.

78. Ibarra C, Jannetta C, Vacanti CA, Cao Y, Kim TH, Upton J, et al. Tissue engineered meniscus: a potential new alternative to allogeneic meniscus transplantation. Transplant Proc. 1997;29(1–2):986–8.

79. Hoben GM, Hu JC, James RA, Athanasiou KA. Self-assembly of fibrochondrocytes and chondrocytes for tissue engineering of the knee meniscus. Tissue Eng. 2007;13(5):939–46.

80. Huey DJ, Athanasiou KA. Maturational growth of self-assembled, functional menisci as a result of TGF-beta1 and enzymatic chondroitinase-ABC stimulation. Biomaterials. 2011;32(8):2052–8.

81. Hoenig E, Winkler T, Mielke G, Paetzold H, Schuettler D, Goepfert C, et al. High amplitude direct compressive strain enhances mechanical properties of scaffold-free tissue-engineered cartilage. Tissue Eng Part A. 2011;17(9–10):1401–11.

82. Mueller SM, Shortkroff S, Schneider TO, Breinan HA, Yannas IV, Spector M. Meniscus cells seeded in type I and type II collagen-GAG matrices in vitro. Biomaterials. 1999;20(8):701–9.

83. Chiari C, Koller U, Kapeller B, Dorotka R, Bindreiter U, Nehrer S. Different behavior of meniscal cells in collagen II/I, III and Hyaff-11 scaffolds in vitro. Tissue Eng Part A. 2008;14(8):1295–304.

84. Ballyns JJ, Gleghorn JP, Niebrzydowski V, Rawlinson JJ, Potter HG, Maher SA, et al. Image-guided tissue engineering of anatomically shaped implants via MRI and micro-CT using injection molding. Tissue Eng Part A. 2008;14(7):1195–202.

85. Baker BM, Nathan AS, Huffman GR, Mauck RL. Tissue engineering with meniscus cells derived from surgical debris. Osteoarthritis Cartilage. 2009;17(3):336–45.

86. Baker BM, Gee AO, Metter RB, Nathan AS, Marklein RA, Burdick JA, et al. The potential to improve cell infiltration in composite fiber-aligned electrospun scaffolds by the selective removal of sacrificial fibers. Biomaterials. 2008;29(15):2348–58.

87. Ionescu LC, Lee GC, Garcia GH, Zachry TL, Shah RP, Sennett BJ, et al. Maturation state-dependent alterations in meniscus integration: implications for scaffold design and tissue engineering. Tissue Eng Part A. 2011;17(1–2):193–204.

88. Ionescu LC, Lee GC, Huang KL, Mauck RL. Growth factor supplementation improves native and engineered meniscus repair in vitro. Acta Biomater. 2012;8(10):3687–94.

89. Fairbank TJ. Knee joint changes after meniscectomy. J Bone Joint Surg Br. 1948;30B(4):664–70.

90. Petty CA, Lubowitz JH. Does arthroscopic partial meniscectomy result in knee osteoarthritis? A systematic review with a minimum of 8 years' follow-up. Arthroscopy. 2011;27(3):419–24.

91. Zaffagnini S, Marcheggiani Muccioli GM, Bulgheroni P, Bulgheroni E, Grassi A, Bonanzinga T, et al. Arthroscopic collagen meniscus implantation for partial lateral meniscal defects: a 2-year minimum follow-up study. Am J Sports Med. 2012;40(10):2281–8.

92. Stone KR, Steadman JR, Rodkey WG, Li ST. Regeneration of meniscal cartilage with use of a collagen scaffold. Analysis of preliminary data. J Bone Joint Surg Am. 1997;79(12):1770–7.

Christos D. Photopoulos and Peter R. Kurzweil

Abbreviations

LCL   Lateral collateral ligament
MCL   Medial collateral ligament

Introduction

The menisci are integral components in maintaining the biomechanics and function of the knee. Interposed between the femoral condyles and the tibial plateau, these paired fibrocartilaginous structures serve in load transmission, shock absorption, proprioception, and stability [1–5]. Historically, tears lead to complete or partial resection of the meniscus. Several studies have since revealed the sequelae of meniscal compromise, including chondral degeneration and predictable arthritis [3]. This consequent increase in awareness of the importance of the menisci has resulted in the push for meniscal preservation. The notion of repairing the meniscus, however, is not a new one, as this was first described by Annandale in 1885 [6]. Since that time, the body of literature on the surgical treatment of meniscal tears has grown immensely. With the advent of arthroscopic surgery, as well as with the development of different techniques and devices, the last three decades have witnessed a tremendous increase in the number of meniscal repairs performed. As the options and technology available for treatment continue to evolve, so too will the indications for repair. The goal of this chapter is to provide a comprehensive overview of meniscal repair: indications will be reviewed, a historical perspective on the evolution of repair will be provided, and the different operative techniques will be presented in detail.

Indications

Evaluating a patient with knee pain begins with a comprehensive history and physical examination. When a meniscal tear is diagnosed, the decision between pursuing a nonoperative course versus an operative course relies on several factors. Indications for surgically addressing tears include: (1) symptoms that affect activities of daily living; (2) physical findings of joint line pain, restricted or painful range of motion; (3) mechanical symptoms such as locking, catching, clicking, and pain with provocative maneuvers; and (4) symptoms recalcitrant to nonoperative modalities [7].

Once the patient is deemed a candidate for operative intervention, the next step is to decide whether to pursue meniscal resection or surgical repair. Indications for repair vary amongst surgeons

C.D. Photopoulos, M.D. (✉)
Hospital of the University of Pennsylvania,
Philadelphia, PA, USA
e-mail: christos.photopoulos@uphs.upenn.edu

P.R. Kurzweil, M.D.
Memorial Orthopaedic Surgical Group, Long Beach,
CA, USA

and are elaborated in a later chapter. However, as a basic principle, every effort must be made to preserve the meniscus in the young, active population. In addition to patient age and level of activity, suitability for meniscal repair relies on several intrinsic factors. These include: tear etiology, location, vascularity, chronicity, configuration, as well as concomitant injuries [8–12]. When all these factors are taken into consideration, the indications for meniscal repair can become more clearly discerned.

Positioning, Diagnostic Arthroscopy, and Meniscal Preparation

Meniscal repair begins with a diagnostic arthroscopy. Despite advanced imaging techniques, direct visualization of the tear and intra-articular environment familiarizes the surgeon with the nuances of the patient's pathology.

As described in previous chapters, positioning begins with the patient in a supine position on a standard operating table. A nonsterile tourniquet is applied to the proximal thigh, but is typically not inflated during the case. This is especially critical when evaluating the vascularity of the tear site. The extremity can then be placed in a well-padded leg holder, which secures the extremity above the knee. This affords circumferential access to the joint while its constraint permits better leverage and thus access to medial, lateral, and posterior aspects of the knee. Other surgeons may prefer to use just a lateral thigh post, which facilitates access to the medial and lateral compartments with valgus pressure and the figure-4 position, respectively. After prepping and draping the patient, portal placement is marked, and the standard anteromedial and anterolateral portals are created. A 4 mm 30° arthroscope is typically used. A 2.9 mm arthroscope, by virtue of its diminished diameter, is also sometimes preferred for better visualization posteriorly.

Although most tears can be seen with the scope in the usual anterolateral portal, sometimes it is best to switch the arthroscope to the anteromedial portal to better visualize the anterior portion of the lateral meniscus. Also, in order to effect adequate visualization in knees with tight medial compartments, surgical partial release of the MCL may be warranted. This can be performed via "outside-in" trephination of the ligament origin using a spinal needle, "inside-out" perforation with an awl or spinal needle, or even via arthroscopic thermal release.

Once the diagnostic arthroscopy is complete, attention is redirected to the meniscal tear. A small probe is inserted into the joint to help better elucidate the tear configuration. In vertical tears, the probe tip can be gently placed inside the tear to help delineate the extent of the tear. Likewise, the upper and lower surfaces of the menisci can be probed to help better visualize horizontal cleavage tears which otherwise could be missed.

Meniscal tear preparation is much like bony fracture nonunion repair. Vascularity must be evaluated, the tear must be reduced, and stable fixation must be applied. Compromise at any one of these steps may hinder the overall success of the repair. To debride the tear edges, a small shaver (without suction) or a small rasp can be used. Cleaning of these edges not only enhances visualization but also promotes a healing response that will serve to further augment the repair [13].

Fixation

Meniscal repair techniques rely on the use of suture or meniscal fixators. Regardless of technique, several basic principles must be considered. It is important that fixation is achieved in a perpendicular fashion across the tear site. This more aptly reduces the tear components, and maximizes the compressive forces across the tear. The stability of fixation is also dependent on the suture configuration. The preferred method of suture fixation is vertical mattress, as studies have shown that this method is biomechanically superior to horizontal mattress techniques [14]. The preferred spacing between fixation points is 5–8 mm, though this depends on the length and stability of the tear. Lastly, after fixation, the knee should be ranged to full flexion and extension. Stressing the fixation site in this fashion allows the surgeon to better evaluate the stability of the construct. Should any gapping or displacement be noted, further fixation or different techniques should be considered.

Techniques to perform a meniscus repair have evolved considerably. The first repairs were performed openly with direct suturing of peripheral tears performed extracapsularly. This practice has largely become abandoned, given the morbidity and compromised visualization. Subsequently, orthopedic surgeons have witnessed the evolution of myriad meniscal repair techniques. Commonly used techniques can be categorized into three groups, each with their own advantages and disadvantages. These include: (1) inside-out repair, (2) outside-in repair, and (3) all-inside repair. Ultimately, the choice of technique is based on tear location, size, configuration, and surgeon preference.

Inside-Out Repair

The first technique for repair is the inside-out repair and was popularized Scott et al in 1986 [7, 15]. This technique involves the arthroscopically guided passage of suture through a cannula from inside the joint capsule, across the meniscal tear, with final retrieval through a carefully dissected counterincision. Retractors in these incisions, such as sterile spoons, commercial retractors, and even small gynecologic specula help protect the neurovascular structures and are well suited for this purpose. The inside-out repair is most suited for middle or posterior tears, and it allows for precise tear reduction and repair. It has traditionally become the gold-standard for repair of most meniscal tears, and still remains the technique of choice for many orthopedic surgeons, especially in parts of the world which cannot support the added expense of meniscal fixators. Additionally, it may be particularly useful in chronically displaced "bucket handle" tears where appreciable force may be necessary to reduce and maintain anatomic position of the meniscus.

A posteromedial counterincision is utilized when repairing medial meniscal tears (Fig. 7.1a). The major structure at risk with this approach is the saphenous nerve, a major cutaneous branch of the femoral nerve. The two divisions of the saphenous nerve are the sartorial and infrapatellar branches, which provide sensation to the anterior and medial aspect of the knee. It is important to note that the relationship of the saphenous nerve to the knee is a dynamic one: the nerve the joint line posteriorly to the posteromedial corner of the knee when the knee is held in flexion, and anteriorly when it is held in extension. Techniques such as the transillumination method can be utilized to avoid injury to the nerve. With the operating room lights dimmed, the medial compartment of the knee can be illuminated

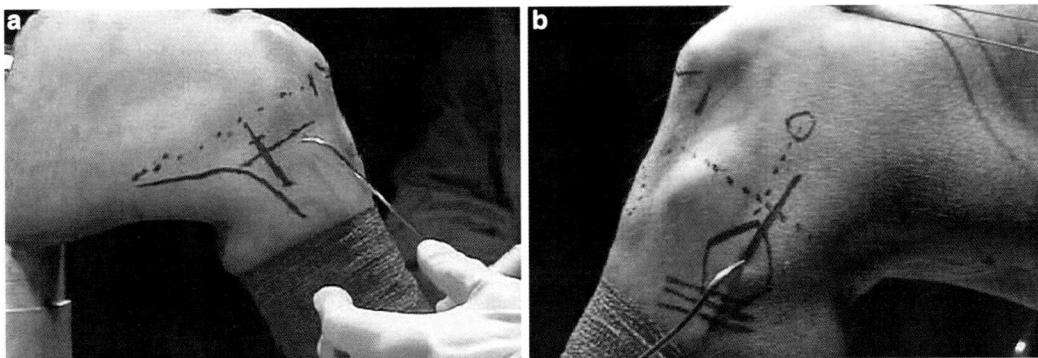

Fig. 7.1 Inside-out repair: (**a**) the posteromedial counterincision is created perpendicular to the knee joint line and just posterior to the MCL and anterior the saphenous nerve; (**b**) posterolateral counterincision is created perpendicular to the joint line and just posterior to the LCL. (*Reprinted from Johnson D, Weiss B: Meniscal repair using the inside-out suture technique. Sports Med Arthrosc. 2012 Jun;20(2): 68–76, with permission from Wolters Kluwer Health*)

a   b   c   d

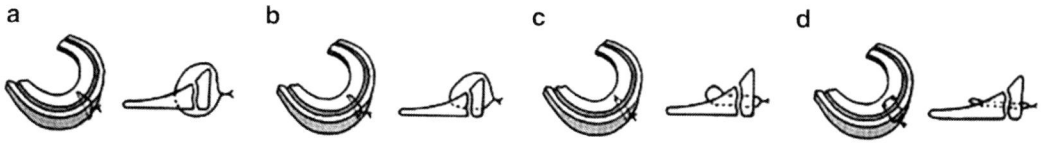

Fig. 7.2 Variations in meniscal suture configuration: (**a–c**) vertical configurations; (**d**) horizontal mattress configuration. (*Modified from Farng E, Sherman O: Meniscal* *repair devices: A clinical and biomechanical literature review. Arthroscopy. 2004 Mar;20(3):273–8, with permission from Elsevier*)

using the arthroscope. A linear shadow that appears represents the saphenous vein; immediately posterior to this lies the saphenous nerve. The posteromedial exposure begins with identifying the joint line with the knee held in 45° of flexion. The posterior border of the superficial medial collateral ligament serves as a landmark for the incision. A 4–5 cm longitudinal incision is developed in line with the posteromedial border of the tibia, just posterior to the MCL. One-third of the incision should extend proximally to the joint, and two thirds should extend distally. Superficial dissection is then taken down through the subcutaneous tissues and carried down to the sartorius fascia. A 4 cm vertical incision is then made through the sartorius fascia, parallel and posterior to the superficial MCL. Bluntly, a fingertip is used to help define the interval interposed between the anterior edge of the pes anserinus muscles and the posterior border of the superficial MCL. A popliteal retractor is then used to retract the sartorius, gracilis, and semitendinosus muscles posteriorly. The medial head of the gastrocnemius is visualized, palpated, and peeled off the capsular tissue, thus exposing the posteromedial capsule.

With lateral meniscal repairs, the principal structure at risk when creating the posterolateral counterincision is the common peroneal nerve (Fig. 7.1b). This approach begins with palpating the joint line and the lateral collateral ligament. A vertical, 4–5 cm incision is created parallel to and just posterior to LCL. Again, one-third of the incision should be proximal to the joint line, and two-thirds should be distal. Dissection is carried down to the fascia of the iliotibial band. The fibular head is then palpated followed by identification of the anterior edge of the biceps femoris, which inserts broadly atop the head of the fibula.

Defining the location of the biceps tendon is of utmost importance, as the common peroneal nerve lies just posteriorly. Once the location of the biceps femoris and iliotibial band is confirmed, the dissection is continued in the soft spot at the posterolateral joint line in the interval between the iliotibial band and biceps tendon. A retractor is placed within this interval, retracting the biceps posteriorly and ensuring protection of the common peroneal nerve. The lateral collateral ligament as well as the lateral head of the gastrocnemius becomes visualized, and the interval between the gastrocnemius and the capsule is then developed. A scalpel is used to perforate the thin fascia that lies laterally to the gastrocnemius tendon. Bluntly, a finger is inserted through this perforation, and the lateral gastrocnemius muscle is gently freed from the posterolateral capsule. A retractor is then placed in this interval, thereby retracting the lateral head of the gastrocnemius, the biceps femoris, and the common peroneal posteriorly, and thus giving exposure to the posterolateral capsule.

Once the desired counterincision is created, suture can be passed into the joint through the contralateral working portal in a variety of different configurations (Fig. 7.2). A single-barreled cannula is used to direct passage of the suture and to facilitate tear reduction. Meticulous attention must always be paid to the cannula once in the joint, as the sharp tips used for meniscal purchase can cause damage to the articular cartilage. Nonabsorbable 2.0 suture, such as Tevdek (Deknatel, Mansfield, MA) or Ticron (Covidien, Mansfield, MA) is preferred, and newer super-strength sutures like OrthoCord (Depuy Mitek, Raynham, MA) and FiberWire (Arthrex, Naples, FL) can also be used. Delivery is accomplished via double-armed needles or reuseable nitinol needles.

The first limb of the suture is passed across the tear as an assistant holding the retractor in the counterincision retrieves the exiting needle. The cannula is then repositioned to create the desired repair configuration (vertical, horizontal, or hybridization) and the second arm of the suture is passed in a similar fashion. The needles are cut off, and a hemostat is used to tag each suture pair. The process is repeated, typically spacing sutures about 5 mm, until the repair is stable. Once all sutures are passed, the suture limbs are tensioned and the fixation is evaluated arthroscopically. When satisfied, the sutures are tied extracapsularly, verifying through direct visualization that no vital structures become imbricated within the knots.

Outside-In Repair

The outside- in technique was developed as a means of minimizing the chance of neurovascular injury that was often seen with inside-out repairs [7]. First described by Warren et al in 1985, this arthroscopically guided technique involves the percutaneous passage of suture into the joint through a cannulated needle placed across the tear [16, 17]. The suture is subsequently retrieved through a second needle, and final fixation is performed extracapsularly via a small portal-sized counterincision. It is most suited for repairing anterior horn tears and middle third tears, and advantages of this method stem from the fact that it is simple, minimally invasive, and inexpensive [18, 19].

There are variations in outside-in repair technique. In its most simple form, all that is required is an 18-gauge needle, suture, and an arthroscopic grasper [20] (Fig. 7.3). Simple "Mulberry Knots" can be created using absorbable suture; however, the authors favor the creation of a vertical mattress configuration. A small needle is percutaneously inserted at the joint line across the tear. If the location is satisfactory, then a small portal like incision is made. First, a 15 blade is used to open the skin and then a hemostat is used to spread down to the capsule. An 18-gauge needle is preloaded with a long (40 cm) suture, either braided or mono-filament, making sure that approximately 10 cm of the suture extends passed the tip of the needle. This will affect a loop when the meniscal tissue is penetrated. While visualizing the tear through the contralateral portal, the needle is passed from the new portal into the joint percutaneously. It should cross the inner and outer rim of the tear, making sure that it ultimately exits the superior surface of the inner rim. A probe can be used to aid in reduction of the tear during passage of the needle while keeping the inner rim from being pushed away from the needle. Once the needle is passed, a grasper is used to grab the created loop of suture at the meniscal inner rim. The needle is then carefully removed from the joint, unloading the remaining suture, making sure not to pull the suture loop from the joint. The 18-gauge needle is then reinserted along the same portal, this time perforating just the outer meniscal rim and again exiting across the superior meniscal surface. This needle should be directed so that it perforates the meniscus to create a vertical or oblique mattress configuration. A separate suture is then passed through the needle and into the joint. A grasper is inserted in the ipsilalteral portal and directed through the loop of the first suture to grab the protruding limb of the second suture. The needle is carefully removed and then the suture is delivered out of the ipsilateral portal. The suture creating the loop is pulled out of the joint, and in effect, the second suture is shuttled through the path of the first insertion, thereby creating a vertical mattress configuration with the second suture. The suture is then tied under arthroscopic visualization to ensure proper tension on the knots.

Commercial kits, such as the Meniscus Mender II (Smith and Nephew Endoscopy, Andover, MA), have also become available for outside-in techniques. With this repair system, two needles are again placed in and outside-to in fashion across the desired sites of fixation. Wire loop stylets are then inserted into the needles. Suture is introduced into the joint via the ipsilateral anterior portal and subsequently fed through one of the loops. The loop stylet is pulled back, capturing the suture, and the loop and needle are carefully removed from the joint. The process is repeated again for the free suture limb within the

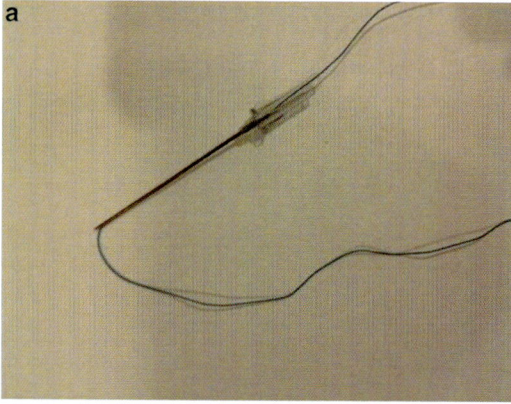
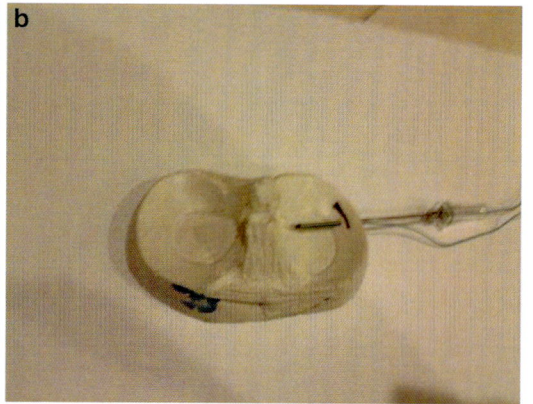
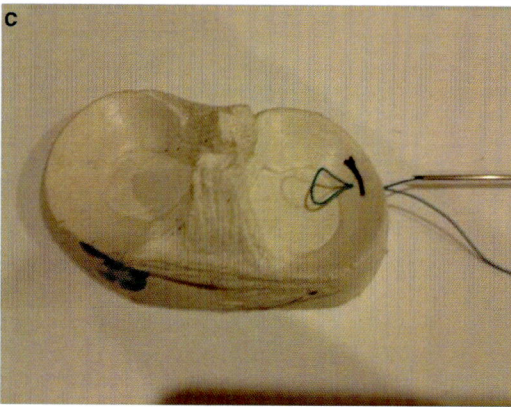
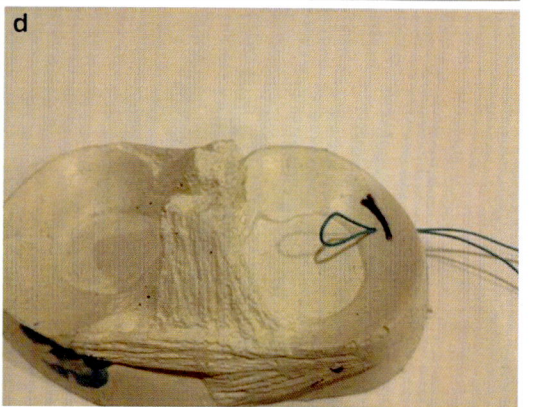
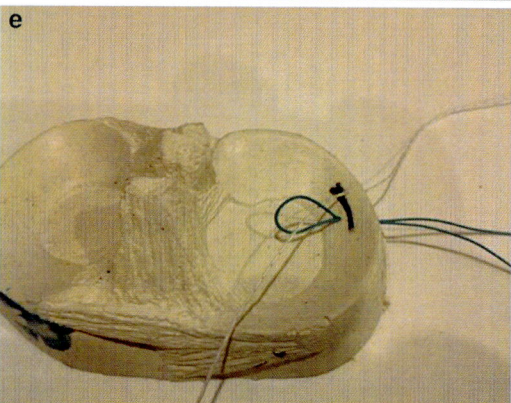
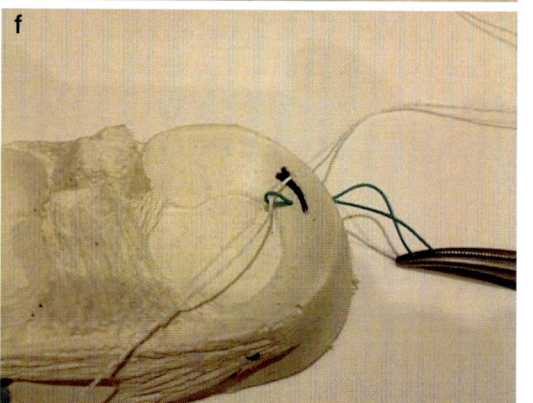
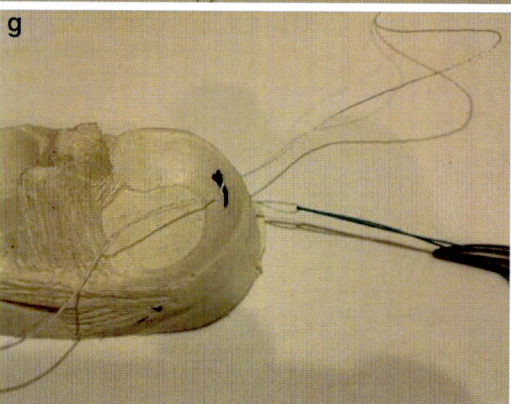
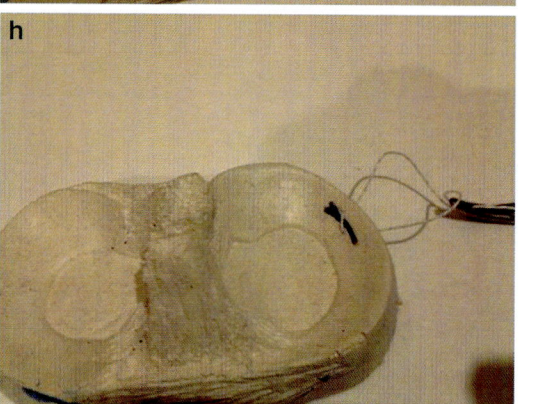

joint. A knot is similarly tied down extracapsularly using a small portal-sized counterincision.

Smaller counterincisions in the outside-in technique have minimized risk to the neurovascular structures. However, these neurovascular structures must be respected: the common peroneal nerve in the lateral aspect of the knee and the saphenous nerve/vein in the medial aspect. The outside-in technique has proven to be successful in the tears of anterior meniscal tears; however, it is more difficult for tears in the posterior horns of the menisci.

All-Inside Repair

The all-inside repair, otherwise known as the "all-arthroscopic" technique, was first introduced to the field of orthopaedics by Morgan et al in 1991 [21]. In this study, the authors utilized posterior accessory portals and suture hooks to shuttle absorbable suture through posterior horn meniscal tears. Subsequent all-inside techniques obviated the need for posterior portals by using meniscal fixators. The orthopedic world has since seen the rapid evolution of the all-inside repair, from rigid devices with barbs to suture-based configurations that allow tensioning after when inserting. Owing to their ease of use, decreased operative time, and lesser risk to neurovascular structures, these all-arthroscopic meniscal fixators have revolutionized the way in which meniscal repairs are performed. Furthermore, newer generations afford pull out strength comparable to inside-out repairs [22–25].

The evolution of fixators came about as a response to the difficulties that arose with the first-generation suture hooks. Many orthopedic surgeons found the tools to be cumbersome and the technique technically demanding [26].

Additionally, given the necessity of creating accessory, posterior portals for passage of instruments, the neurovascular structures were still deemed to be at risk. Thus, the second generation of constructs relied on the use "suture anchors"—implants placed across the tear and affixed along the outer meniscal rim. One such device is the T-fix (Smith & Nephew), an implant comprised of a 3 mm polyethylene bar connected to a 2.0 braided suture at its midpoint. Using a spinal needle, the implant is delivered across the meniscal tear, and to the other surface of the meniscus. A second anchor is passed and deployed adjacent to the first anchor, and a knot pusher is used to tie the two sutures arthroscopically. This technique represented the first all-inside suture technique that did not require the use of any accessory portals. Though results from use of the T-Fix were favorable, the desire for improved compression paved the way for the next generation of fixators [26].

The next wave of implant evolution relied on the use of what became known as "compression-type" design. Common devices in this third-generation all-inside implant category are the well-known meniscal arrows, screws, darts, and staples (Fig. 7.4). These biodegradable fixators function as tac-like implants that are either screwed or pushed into place in order to reduce and affix the inner rim of the meniscus to the outer rim. Due to their ease of use, their appearance on the market was met with initial enthusiasm. However, later developments exposed the complications of this technique. Implants tended to be too rigid, tended to become proud, either by initial technique or subsequent loosening, and were found to cause femoral condylar "grooving" and consequent chondral injury. Additionally, several reports arose citing inflammatory reactions to the implants have caused them to largely fall out of favor [26]. Although deemed absorbable,

Fig. 7.3 Outside-in repair: (**a**) An 18-gauge needle is loaded with suture, ensuring that 10 cm extends passed the needle tip. (**b**) The needle is inserted across the tear, crossing the inner and outer rim. (**c**) The needle is carefully pulled back. (**d**) An intra-articular suture loop is created. (**e**) A separate suture is reinserted across the outer meniscal rim and through the previous suture loop. (**f**) A hemostat is used to pull the suture loop from the joint. (**g**) The suture loops is completely withdrawn. (**h**) A vertical mattress configuration is created

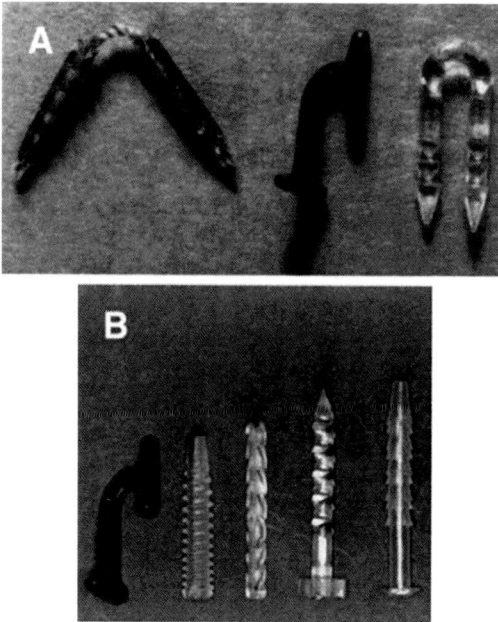

Fig. 7.4 All-inside repair: third-generation fixators: (**a**) (*left* to *right*) SDsorb Staple, Meniscal Repair System, Biomet Staple; (**b**) Clearfix Screw, Arthrex Dart, Bionx Meniscus Arrow, Linvatec Biostinger (*Modified from Farng E, Sherman O: Meniscal repair devices: A clinical and biomechanical literature review. Arthroscopy. 2004 Mar;20(3):273–8, with permission from Elsevier*)

the dissolution rate was very slow and the risk of articular damage was protracted [27, 28].

Given the drawbacks of the previous generations, the fourth and most current generation of all-inside meniscal repair implants followed. These suture based implants incorporate dual anchors connected by a pre-tied, sliding, self-locking knot, thus permitting variable tensioning across the tear. Their introduction to the joint and their tensioning is done entirely arthroscopically, and no accessory portals or implant entry sites

are required. The two prototypical implants initially introduced to the market were the FasT-Fix (Smith and Nephew) and the RapidLoc (Depuy Mitek, Raynham, MA).

Several fourth-generation all-inside implants are currently available. One commonly used repair system is the FAST-FIX 360 (Smith & Nephew) (Fig. 7.5a). This implant is comprised of two 5 mm polymer anchors connected by a pre-tied 2.0 nonabsorbable polyethylene suture. A delivery needle containing the implant is inserted into the joint by use of a slotted cannula. The curved tip of the needle must be pointing towards the cannula as it is introduced into the joint, thus preventing inadvertent injury to the femoral articular surfaces. The needle is carefully positioned on the superior border of the outer meniscal rim, and the first anchor is deployed across the meniscus. The delivery needle is then carefully retracted, leaving the first anchor at the menisco-capsular periphery to function as a "backstop." The second anchor is then deployed across the inner rim in a similar fashion. The delivery needle is then removed from the joint, and the suture is tensioned to reduce the tear. A tensioning suture-cutting device can be inserted to facilitate with reduction. The knot is then cut once adequate reduction is achieved. Other commercial systems utilizing this dual anchor backstop technology are also available. Depuy Mitek has replaced the RapidLoc implant with the newer OmniSpan system, an implant preloaded with two PEEK (Polyether ether ketone) backstops connected by pre-tied 2-0 OrthoCord suture (Fig. 7.5b). As in the FAST-FIX 360, anchor deployment and suture tensioning is performed via a single inserter and a trigger grip handle. The success of these fourth-generation

Fig. 7.5 All-inside repair, fourth-generation backstop fixators: (**a**) FAST-FIX 360 (Smith & Nephew) (i) Implant, (ii) Instruments, (iii) A slotted canula is inserted into the joint to help guide the passage of the delivery needle, (iv) The delivery needle containing the implant is inserted across the meniscal tear and the "backstop" is deployed, (v) The needle is retracted and a reinserted at another location to obtain the desired suture configuration, (vi) The needle is removed from the joint and the needle is tensioned to reduce the tear. (**b**) OmniSpan (Depuy Mitek) (**a**(i), **b** *reprinted from Barber FA, Herbert MA, Bava ED, Drew OR: Biomechanical testing of suture-based meniscal repair devices containing ultrahigh-molecular weight polyethylene suture: update 2011. Arthroscopy. 2012 June; 28 (6):827–34, with permission from Elsevier*)

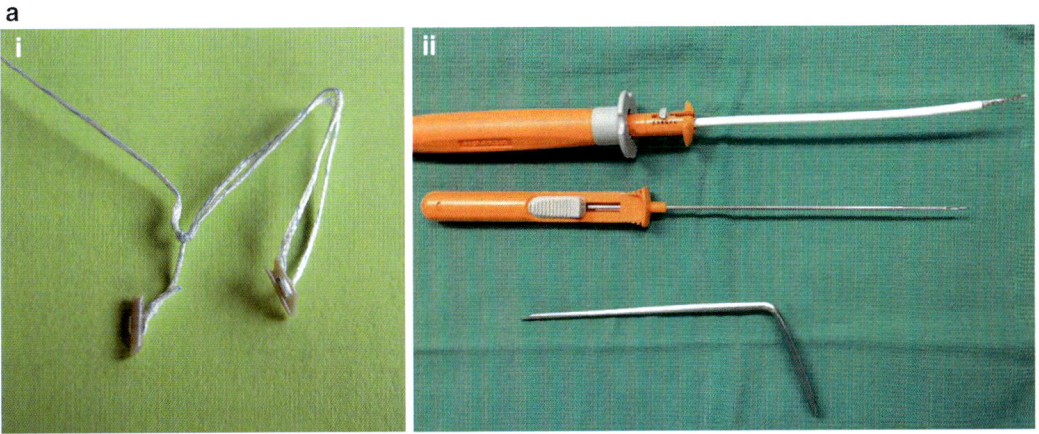

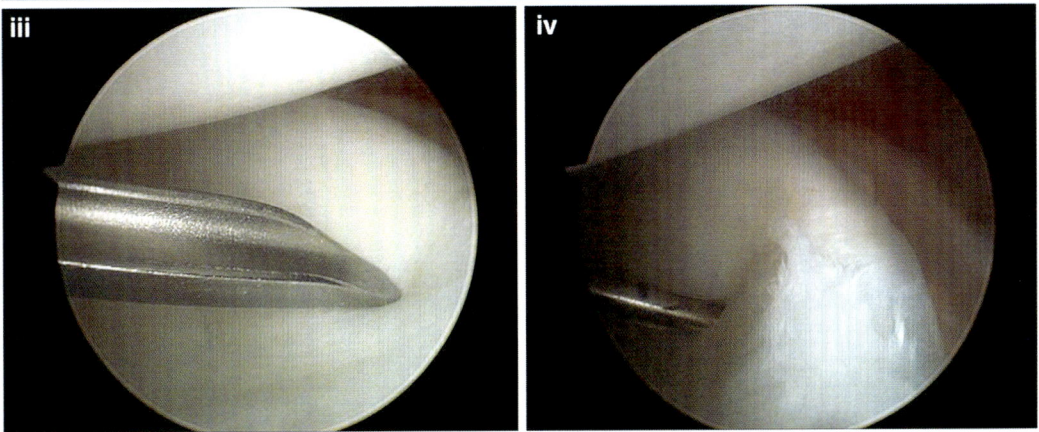

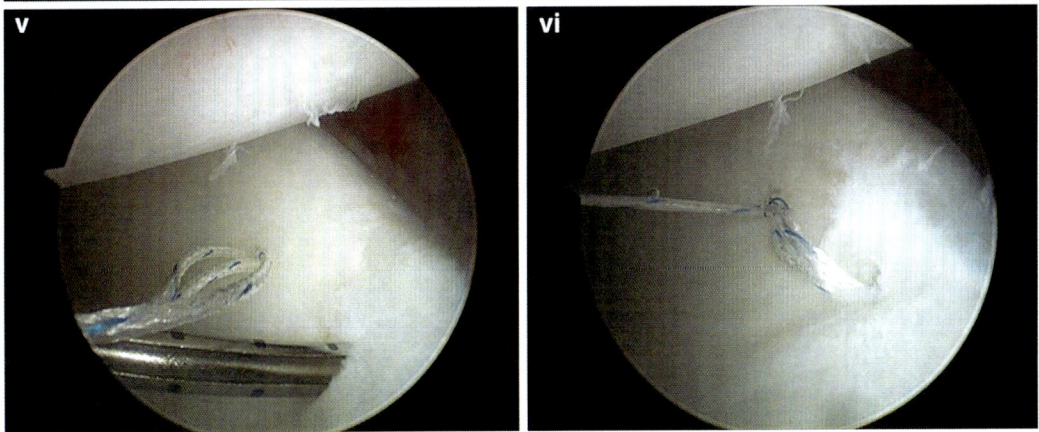

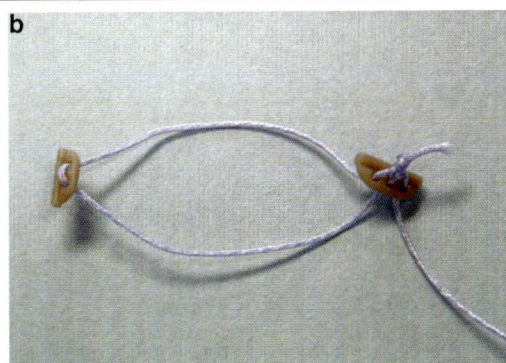

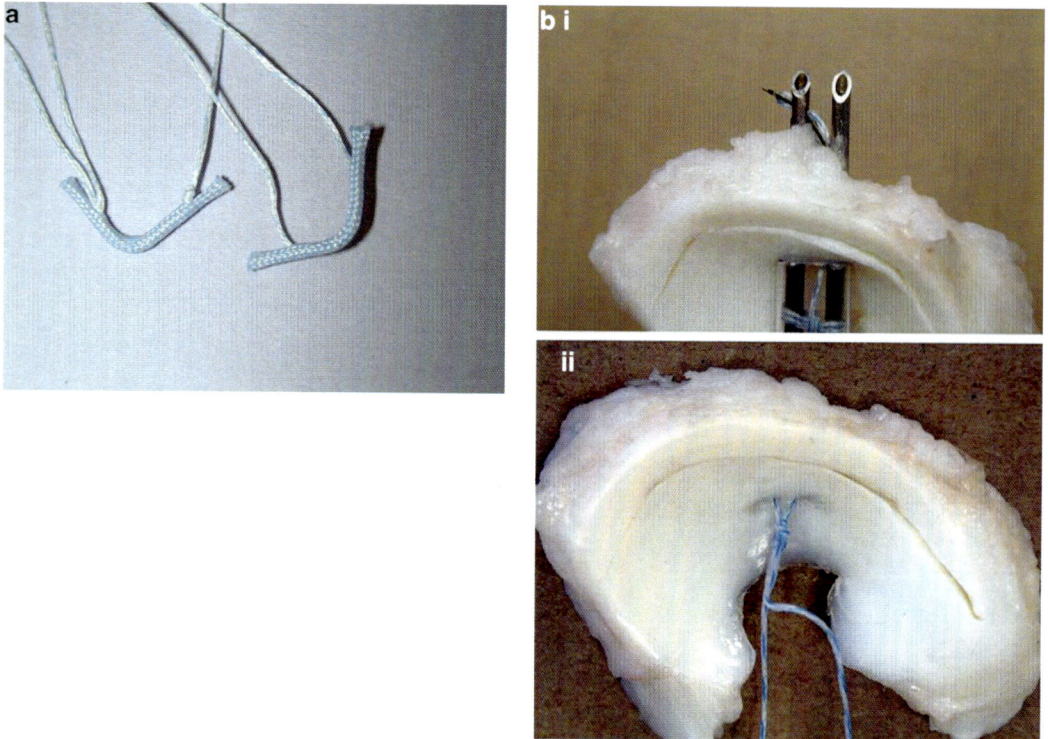

Fig. 7.6 All-inside repair, fourth-generation all-suture fixators: (**a**) MaxFire (Biomet), (**b**) CrossFix II (Cayenne Medical) (i) Instrument insertion, and (ii) Tear reduction and fixation (*Reprinted from Barber FA, Herbert MA,*

Schroeder A, et al: Biomechanical testing of new meniscal repair techniques containing ultra high-molecular weight polyethylene suture. Arthroscopy 25:959–967, 2009 with permission from Elsevier)

repair systems rely on their ease of usage, decreased chondral injury, and versatile application to different parts of the meniscus. Initial studies assessing their long-term success have thus far been promising, with pull-out strength exceeding 100 N—comparable to an inside-out vertical mattress repairs [25].

Recently, all-suture fixators, such as the MaxFire (Biomet, Warsaw, Indiana), have emerged (Fig. 7.6). Similar to the FAST-FIX 360 and the OmniSpan, the MaxFire relies on a dual anchor suture tensioning for fixation. However, suture coils are used as backstops instead of polymer anchors. The latest advent in all-suture implants is the CrossFix II (Cayenne Medical, Scottsdale, AZ), a device that deploys an instantaneous mattress suture without relying on anchors for fixation. With this system, adjacent needles spaced 3 mm apart are incorporated within the delivery device. These needles are

simultaneously inserted across the inner and outer meniscal rims. Once the needle tips extend beyond the periphery of the menisco-capsular junction, a curved crossing-needle containing the 0-polyethylene suture is deployed from one of the delivery needles and automatically captured by the adjacent needle. The delivery needles are then carefully withdrawn from the joint, leaving a 3 mm stitch at the capsular periphery, and a pre-tied Westin slip knot at the meniscal surface. The tear is then reduced by suture tensioning with added half-hitches as necessary.

Although these fourth-generation implants have demonstrated early success, several precautions and limitations must be recognized. Care must be taken during insertion, as plunging to deeply through the capsule can cause neurovascular injury. Depth gauges/stops should be used when possible, and corresponding depth limiter adjustments should be made to the delivery devices prior to insertion. Limitations are governed by price and surgeon preference. Though suitable for many meniscal tears, these fixators generally require a peripheral rim for anchoring and cannot be used for meniscocapsular separations. Likewise, anterior horn tears are often difficult to access and may necessitate the use of alternate techniques.

Conclusion

Over the past several decades, several studies citing the long-term consequences of meniscal damage or loss have enhanced our awareness of the importance of the meniscus to knee integrity and function. When addressing meniscal tears, several factors must be evaluated when considering treatment options. Likewise, when considering repair, several components of the patient's pathology help determine the suitability of repair. Although the concept of meniscal repair has been around since the nineteenth century, it is only in the last three decades that we have witnessed the exponential growth in utilization of these procedures. The indications for meniscal repair are somewhat defined, but continue to evolve. Several studies have illustrated the success of these techniques. However, as methods and implants for meniscal repair continue to be refined, several questions remain unanswered. Longer-term studies are needed to better evaluate the long-term-success rates of more current techniques, and more prospective analyses are needed to better define postoperative rehabilitation algorithms. The future of meniscal repair is a promising one, and with current advents in biologics, tissue engineering, cell-based techniques, and instrument sophistication, the field of meniscal surgery will surely continue to grow.

References

1. Bland-Sutton J. Ligaments: their nature and morphology. 2nd ed. London; 1897.
2. Greis PE, Bardana DD, Holmstrom MC, Burks RT. Meniscal injury: 1. Basic science and evaluation. J Am Acad Orthop Surg. 2002;10(3):168–76.
3. McDermott ID, Amis AA. The consequences of meniscectomy. J Bone Joint Surg Br Vol. 2006;88(12): 1549–56.
4. Walker PS, Erkman MJ. The role of the menisci in force transmission across the knee. Clin Orthop Related Res. 1975;109:184–92.
5. Levy IM, Torzilli PA, Gould JUD, et al. The effect of medial meniscectomy on anterior-posterior motion of the knee. J Bone Joint Surg Am. 1982;64:883–8.
6. Annandale T. An operation for displaced semilunar cartilage. Br Med J. 1885;1(1268):779.
7. Delee J, Drez D, Miller M. DeLee & Drez's orthopaedic sports medicine: principles and practice. 3rd ed. Philadelphia, PA: Elsevier; 2010.
8. Scott WN, editor. Surgery of the knee. 4th ed. Philadelphia, PA: Elsevier; 2006. p. 481–90.
9. Rispoli DM, Miller MD. Options in meniscal repair. Clin Sports Med. 1999;18(1):77–91.
10. Cannon WD, Vittori JM. The incidence of healing in arthroscopic meniscal repairs in anterior cruciate ligament-reconstructed knees versus stable knees. Am J Sports Med. 1992;20(2):176–81.
11. Noyes FR, Barber-Westin SD. Arthroscopic repair of meniscus tears extending into the avascular zone with or without anterior cruciate ligament reconstruction in patients 40 years of age and older. Arthroscopy. 2000; 16(8):822–9.
12. DeHaven KE. Decision-making factors in the treatment of meniscal lesions. Clin Orthop Relat Res. 1990;252:49–54.
13. Ritchie JR, Miller MD, Bents RT, Smith DK. Meniscal repair in the goat model. The use of healing adjuncts and the role of magnetic resonance arthrography in repair evaluation. Am J Sports Med. 1998;26(2): 278–84.
14. Post WR, Akers SR, Kish V. Load to failure of common meniscal repair techniques: effects of suture technique and material. Arthroscopy. 1997;13(6): 731–6.
15. Scott GA, Jolly BL, Henning CE. Combined posterior incision and arthroscopic intra-articular repair of the meniscus: an examination of factors affecting healing. J Bone Joint Surg Am. 1986;68:847–61.
16. Warren RF. Arthroscopic meniscus repair. Arthroscopy. 1985;1:170–2.
17. Rodeo SA, Warren RF. Meniscal repair using the outside-to-inside technique. Clin Sports Med. 1996; 15:469–81.
18. Rodeo SA. Arthroscopic meniscal repair with use of the outside-in technique. Instr Course Lect. 2000;49:195–206.
19. van Trommel MF, Simonian PT, Potter HG, et al. Different regional healing rates with the outside-in technique for meniscal repair. Am J Sports Med. 1998;26:446–52.
20. Laupattarakasem W, Sumanont S, Kesprayura S, Kasemkijwattana C. Arthroscopic outside-in meniscal repair through a needle hole. Arthroscopy. 2004;20(6):654–7.
21. Morgan CD. The "all-inside" meniscus repair. Arthroscopy. 1991;7(1):120–5.

22. Kocabey Y, Chang HC, Brand JC, et al. A biomechanical comparison of the FasT-Fix meniscal repair suture system and the RapidLoc device in cadaver meniscus. Arthroscopy. 2006;22:406–13.

23. Mehta VM, Terry MA. Cyclic testing of 3 all inside meniscal repair devices. Am J Sports Med. 2009; 37(12):2435–9.

24. Barber FA, Herbert MA, Schroeder A, et al. Biomechanical testing of new meniscal repair techniques containing ultra high-molecular weight polyethylene suture. Arthroscopy. 2009;25:959–67.

25. Barber FA, Herbert MA, Bava ED, Drew OR. Biomechanical testing of suture-based meniscal repair devices containing ultrahigh-molecular weight polyethylene suture: update 2011. Arthroscopy. 2012 June;28(6):827–34.

26. Turman KA, Diduch DR, Miller MD. All-inside meniscal repair. Sports Health. 2009;1(5):438–44.

27. Kurzweil PR, Tifford CD, Ignacio EM. Unsatisfactory clinical results of meniscal repair using the meniscus arrow. Arthroscopy. 2005;21(8):905–7.

28. Lee GP, Diduch D. Deteriorating outcomes after meniscal repair using the meniscal arrow in knees undergoing concurrent anterior cruciate ligament reconstruction: increased failure rate with long-term follow-up. Am J Sports Med. 2005;33:1138–41.

Meniscal Posterior Root Tear

8

Amy E. Sewick, Ann Marie Kelly, and John D. Kelly IV

Introduction

While the importance of the menisci to overall knee biomechanics and functioning has long been recognized, further attention is now being directed to the role of the posterior horns of the menisci. Meniscal posterior root tears (MPRT) are becoming increasingly recognized and addressed.

The menisci of the knee are crescent-shaped structures of fibrocartilage composed of collagen bundles arranged in circumferential and radial orientations. The menisci are attached to the tibial plateau both anteriorly and posteriorly. The posterior horn of the medial meniscus is bigger than the anterior horn of the medial meniscus; however, it has a smaller insertion site surface area [1]. The menisci are fixed in place and prevented from extruding by the anterior and posterior attachments, coronary ligaments, as well as the circumferential fibers of the meniscus [2]. This firm fixation affords the meniscus the ability to dissipate axial loads and transfer stress in a radial direction (hoop stress). The most common location

A.E. Sewick, M.D. (✉) • J.D. Kelly IV, M.D.
Department of Orthopaedic Surgery, Hosptial of the University of Pennsylvania, 3400 Spruce Street, 2 Silverstein, Philadelphia, PA 19104, USA
e-mail: asewick@gmail.com

A.M. Kelly
Department of Orthopedics, University of Pennsylvania, 235 South Street, Philadelphia, PA 19104, USA

for medial meniscal injury is the posterior horn [3]. Radial tears of the posterior horn of the medial meniscus are fairly common with the overall prevalence cited as approximately 10% of all meniscal tears and are seen more frequently in patients of Asian descent [4, 5]. Loss of the posterior horn attachment results in extrusion of the meniscus and renders the meniscus essentially useless. Hoop stresses are lost, rendering the remaining meniscus impotent as a means of providing stress shielding to the tibiofemoral articulation [6]. Marzo found that avulsion of the posterior root of the medial meniscus leads to an increase in peak tibiofemoral contact pressure and a decrease in tibiofemoral contact area [7]. A cadaver study by Hein et al. showed that in a mechanically loaded cadaver model, an avulsed medial meniscus had an average medial displacement of 3.28 mm compared to an intact medial meniscus with 1.60mm medial displacement ($p<0.001$) [8]. In addition, this study showed significantly increased gap formation between the medial meniscal root and the medial meniscus in the avulsed state versus the intact or repaired models. Another cadaver study by Allaire et al. showed that following a medial meniscal posterior root tear, there was an increase of 25% in peak contact pressure compared to the intact knee and also showed restoration of peak contact pressures to normal following meniscal root repair [6]. Articular wear as well as joint space narrowing have also been shown to be accelerated following medial meniscal root avulsion [9].

J.D. Kelly IV (ed.), *Meniscal Injuries: Management and Surgical Techniques*,
DOI 10.1007/978-1-4614-8486-8_8, © Springer Science+Business Media New York 2014

Mechanism of Injury

Meniscal root tears are seen both traumatically and as a degenerative process. Risk factors for MMPRT previously described include increased body mass index (BMI), age, varus knees, and female sex [10–12]. A sudden twisting maneuver or deep squat can sufficiently load the posterior horn to create an avulsion. Deep squatting is associated with femoral rollback. The posterior horns of the menisci essentially prevent excessive rollback and help to contain the condyles within the tibiofemoral compartment. Sudden loading, as seen in a forceful squatting maneuver, may create a shear stress to the horn attachment and avulse the posterior horn from its bony insertion.

With age, chronic attritional tears may occur. Rather than pure posterior horn bone avulsions, radial tears approximating the meniscal insertion may develop. The effect on meniscal function is the same as the pure avulsion—loss of hoop stress.

Posterior horn insufficiency is also associated with osteoarthritis. Whether the arthritic manifestations are the result of or the cause of degeneration is a matter of debate. Since the posterior horn of the medial meniscus bears most of the weight-bearing stress of the medial compartment, a "wear and tear" mechanism likely leads to tear evolution [13]. Nonetheless, in the case of mild to moderate degenerative changes, recognition and treatment of posterior horn insufficiency may provide the patient considerable symptomatic relief.

Presentation

Patients with root avulsion usually present with joint line pain. These patients may describe a history of twisting injury. Pain with deep knee flexion is common. Mechanical symptoms including locking, catching, or clicking may be present. As discussed previously, root tears may be part of a degenerative process. Again, it is impossible to determine if the degenerative changes seen accompany the root tear or if they are a *result* of the tear. If the degenerative changes are not advanced, then consideration for repair should be

embraced as a means of protecting the chondral surfaces. Generally, root avulsion tears seem to occur more commonly on the medial side of the knee, likely a result of the increased constraint seen with the medial meniscus. However, a subset of root injury, the partial lateral root tear, is commonly seen with acute ACL injury. These injuries result from the violent shearing that occurs with the pivot shift phenomenon. These tears may or may not require repair, depending on how much horn attachment is left. Shelbourne et al. contend that these lateral posterior horn tears remain stable and do not require surgical fixation [14].

Physical Exam

Patients with meniscal root injury will usually demonstrate a knee effusion and manifest joint line tenderness. Joint line pain with deep squatting or a "duck" walk will usually be present. The Thessaly test, whereupon the patient is asked to twist on a semi-flexed leg, may be positive. Also, the examiner must discern the "degenerative" index of each knee, as imaging findings may only tell half the story. Osteophytes, crepitance, flexion contractures, and Baker's cysts all indicate a knee with more advanced degenerative changes.

Imaging

Standing and 30° PA flexion views are very helpful in assessing chondral wear. MRI is the imaging study of choice to detect root injury. Of note, scanners with 1.5 T strength or greater obviate the need for gadolinium enhancement.

Extrusion of the meniscus on the coronal AP images is perhaps the most characteristic finding of root injury (Fig. 8.1). If the meniscus is extruded more than 3 mm, then a root injury must be suspected. Extrusion may also occur with degeneration of the meniscus, as the worn-out tissues merely lose their secure anchoring properties. However, root injury or avulsion will generally be more displaced than mere degeneration.

On the sagittal MRI images, root injury will manifest with anterior displacement of the meniscus. As the meniscus breaks free of its posterior horn attachment, its tendency is to slide anteriorly, rather than posteriorly. The amount of anterior displacement thus correlates with the degree of posterior horn detachment.

Axial images may reveal separation of the posterior horn and tibia. These "spaces" which enhance on T2 images are often subtle but may significantly reinforce evidence of a root injury.

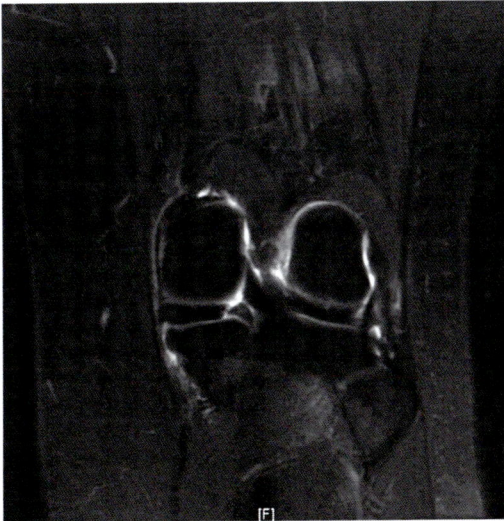

Fig. 8.1 This coronal image shows an extruded medial meniscus

Treatment

If degenerative changes are not pronounced, then repair of meniscal root injury should be considered. The Kellgren-Lawrence scale is helpful in formulating treatment plans. Harner et al. described some contraindications for meniscal root repair: significant medial joint space narrowing and/or Fairbanks changes, diffuse grade 3 or 4 cartilage changes in the articular cartilage of the femoral condyle or tibial plateau, and greater than $3°$ of asymmetric varus alignment [15]. In general, if there is less than 50 % joint space narrowing, the author favors an attempt at repair.

After the patient and surgeon have decided to pursue surgical treatment, the surgeon examines the tear arthroscopically during a diagnostic knee scope. The surgeon must examine the tear characteristics and the tissue quality (Fig. 8.2). In addition, the surgeon should evaluate the articular cartilage of the knee joint. At times, during arthroscopic inspection, the tissues are too poor to support repair, and the arthritis index is greater than anticipated. Otherwise, a properly executed repair presents minimal harm to the patient. After the tear and the surrounding knee structures have been thoroughly evaluated and the decision is made to pursue fixation, then the tear should be debrided to remove any meniscal flaps or fraying that may worsen visualization and/or impede fixation (Fig. 8.3).

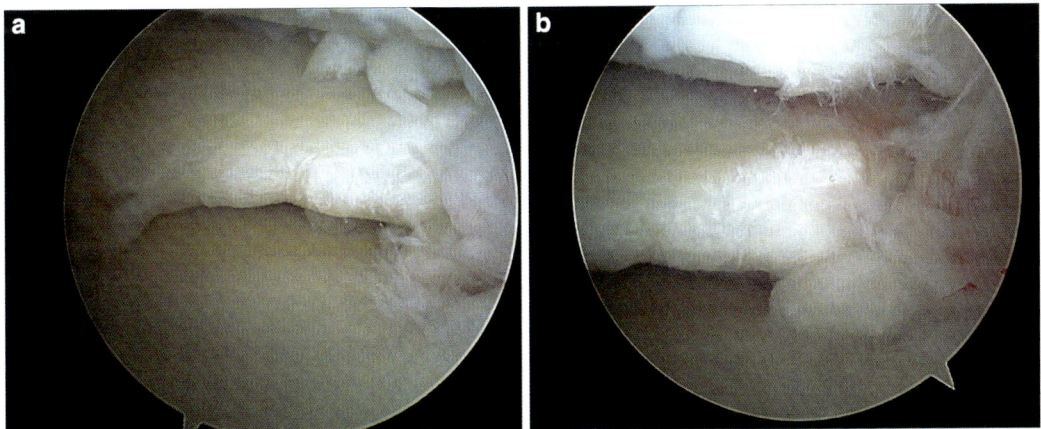

Fig. 8.2 (**a**, **b**) These arthroscopic images demonstrate a root tear of the posterior horn of the medial meniscus

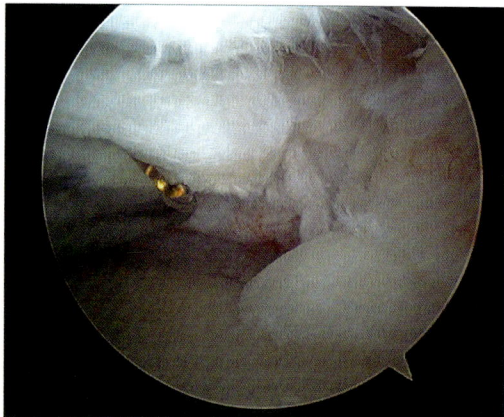

Fig. 8.3 An arthroscopic shaver is used to debride the frayed edges of the tear

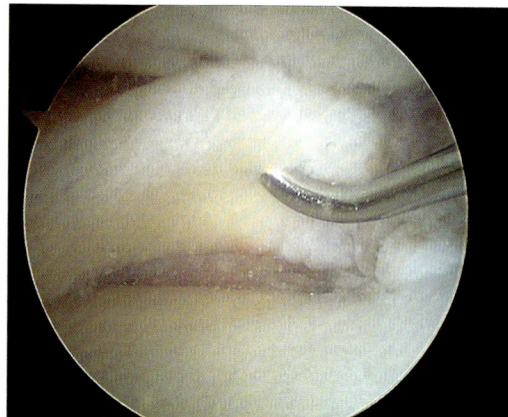

Fig. 8.4 A suture hook is used to pass a shuttle into the posterior horn fragment

Once the tear has been debrided, then an assessment must be made as to which type of repair should be performed. A probe can be used to examine the tear and evaluate tissue quality and extent of the tear (Fig. 8.4). Since the essence of the injury is an avulsion, most repairs require fixation to bone. Rarely, there is enough residual posterior horn tissue to allow a repair using all-inside meniscal fixators (Fig. 8.5a–e) or using a luggage tag technique (Fig. 8.6a–c). In most cases, the tissue will not support suture fixation, and attachment of the avulsed segment to bone is required.

Bone Tunnel Technique

A leg holder is extremely helpful in applying the necessary valgus stress to the knee to open up the medial compartment. For medial injury, a high lateral viewing portal is created and the diagnosis confirmed with probing of the meniscus. A low medial parapatellar portal is established first for probing and later for viewing. Medial portal creation closer to the joint line affords easier access to the posterior horn. A second medial portal is made more medially, just above the joint line, and is necessary for suture shuttling.

In order to execute the surgery readily, release of the medial collateral ligament (MCL) is necessary. This can be performed numerous ways. A simple spinal needle can be used to trephinate the

origin of the MCL. Alternatively, a microfracture awl or spinal needle can be employed from the lateral portal to create small perforations in the meniscocapsular junction. Finally, in especially tight knees, the author favors thermal ablation of the superficial and deep MCL.

To execute repair, the arthroscope is switched to the medial portal, and the contralateral high lateral portal is used to gain suture purchase of the meniscus. The author favors a spectrum 45-degree type suture hook to pierce the meniscus with a PDS suture. The No. 1 PDS is used to shuttle a No. 2 FiberWire (Arthrex, Naples, FL) (Fig. 8.7). The accessory medial portal is used for retrieving during shuttling. After the first suture is passed and shuttled, a second "bite" is then obtained, as perpendicular as possible to the first, with the shuttle steps repeated. It is important to take more than one bite as tissue quality may be suboptimal. Rarely, use of the posteromedial portal, or even a posterior puncture with a spinal needle, may be necessary to pierce the meniscus in an orthogonal fashion. Once both suture limbs are shuttled through the avulsed segment, they are retrieved through the accessory medial portal (Fig. 8.8).

The bone tunnel for suture anchorage must now be created. An ACL guide with a low profile tip is placed via the medial parapatellar portal, while viewing is performed from the lateral portal. Before the tip is placed on the posterior horn insertion, the drill guide location is marked with an electrothermal device. Recall that the posterior horn

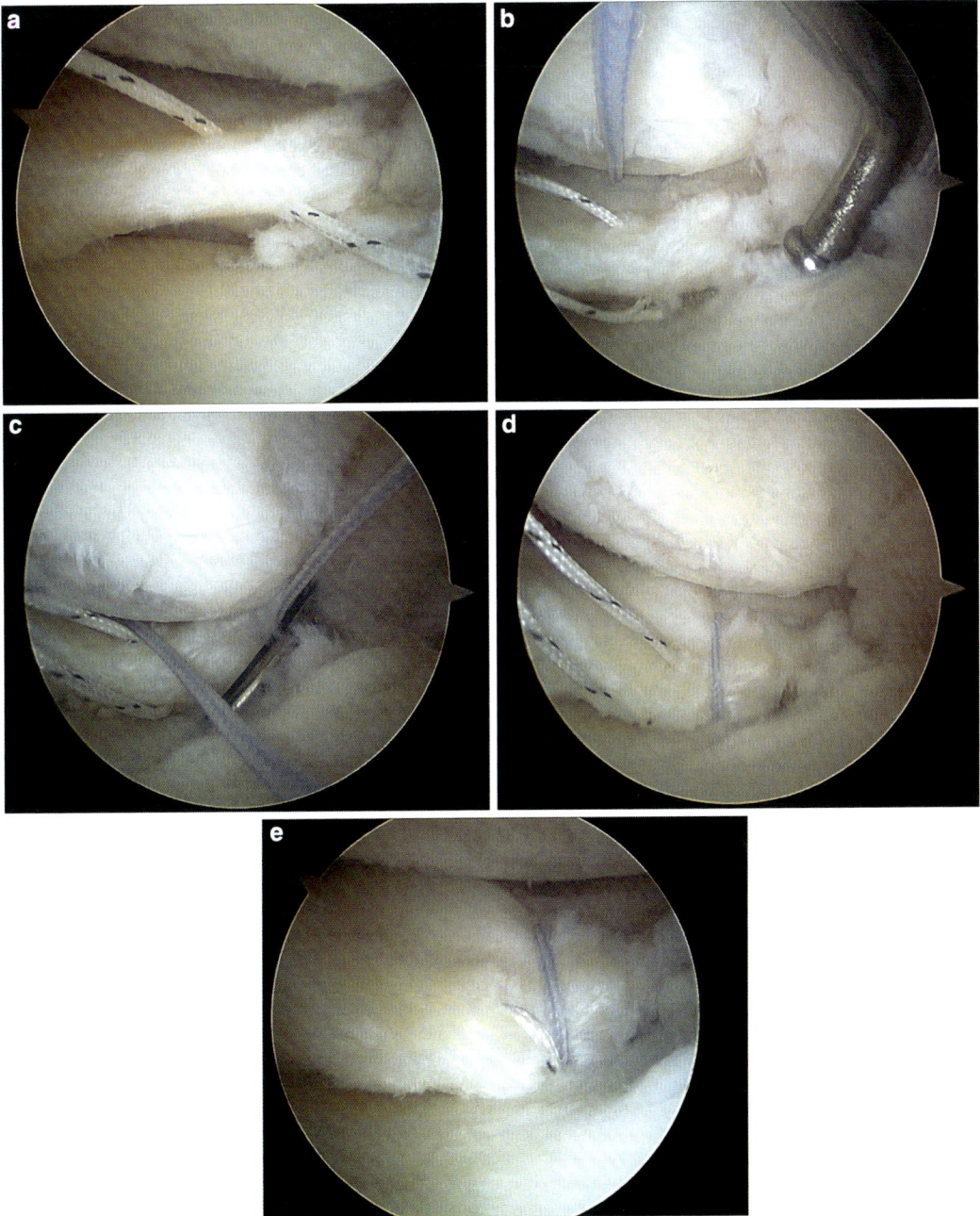

Fig. 8.5 The tissue quality of this meniscus was deemed to be suitable for an all-inside repair. (**a**) The first suture is passed through the tear. (**b**) The second suture is then passed through the tear. (**c**, **d**) The first suture is tied. (**e**) A final image demonstrating the repaired tear

of the medial meniscus is much more posterior than that of the lateral meniscus.

The bullet tip of the drill is applied to the skin overlying the tibia, then the tip is removed, and a small incision is created on the medial tibia down to periosteum. Enough exposure to ensure suture retrieval is attained. The bone tunnel is created with a standard 3/32-in Steinmann pin and the

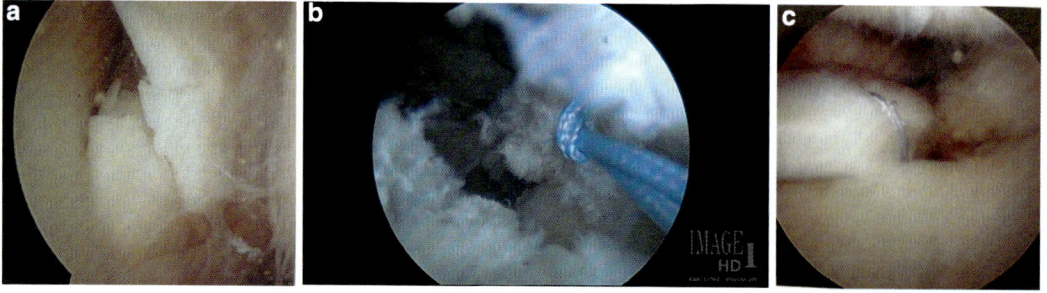

Fig. 8.6 (**a**) This image demonstrates a meniscal root avulsion tear. (**b**) A luggage tag stitch has been thrown through the fragments of avulsed meniscus. (**c**) The avulsed meniscus is now repaired

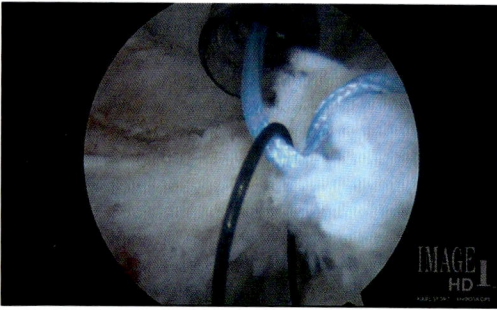

Fig. 8.7 No. 1 PDS is used to shuttle FiberWire through the avulsed meniscus

drill "bullet" is firmly applied to the bone surface. Marking the tip of the Steinmann pin with marker ink helps locate the drill tunnel when the pin is removed. A Hewson suture passer is immediately threaded into the tunnel through the bullet to retrieve the first pair of sutures.

A lobster-claw-type instrument is passed from the lateral portal through the Hewson suture passer and then used to retrieve two suture limbs from the accessory medial portal. The suture passer is withdrawn and the sutures are clamped. A lobster-claw device is applied around the sutures to ensure easy discernment of the tunnel for the second "pass" of the Hewson device. The remaining pair is passed in similar fashion and tied to a plastic or titanium button with the knee in nearly full extension.

Suture Anchor Technique

A suture anchor may be inserted from a high posteromedial portal. While viewing through the

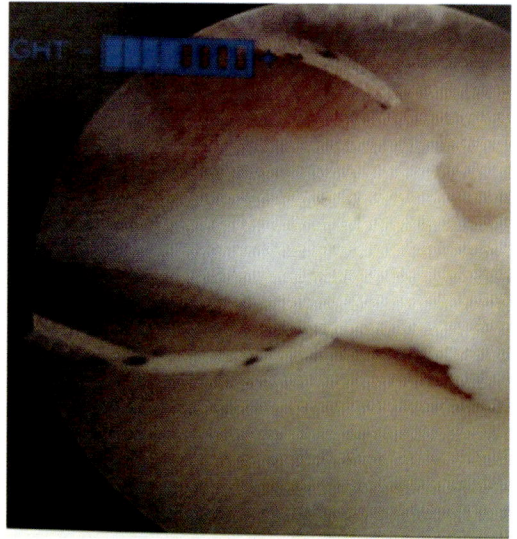

Fig. 8.8 A FiberWire has now been passed through the avulsed meniscus

Gilquist portal (through the notch), a 70-degree scope may be helpful but is not necessary. Alternatively, a high posterolateral portal may be employed for anchor insertion; however, this requires the use of the "transseptal portal" as described by Kim et al. [16]. Practitioners unfamiliar with transseptal portal creation are encouraged to practice this technique in the lab, as there is indeed a steep learning curve.

Once the anchor is placed, the suture limbs must be shuttled through the meniscal tissue. This is best accomplished with suture hooks and shuttling of PDS suture. While viewing through the notch, the suture limbs are retrieved via a cannula placed in the posteromedial portal. A larger (at least 7 mm) size cannula is necessary to afford room for the suture hooks. The suture limbs may be shuttled via the cannula or via an accessory posteromedial portal, located proximal to the first. Once suture limbs are shuttled through tissue, they are tied from the posteromedial cannula.

For the more challenging transseptal portal technique, one may view from the posterolateral portal while retrieving and shuttling is executed from one or two posteromedial portals.

Rehabilitation

Unlike standard meniscal repair, where weight-bearing in extension may be permissible, root repairs require strict adherence to a reduced weight-bearing protocol. Weight-bearing in extension will tax the security of the repair and stress the root attachment. Furthermore, since femoral "rollback" does indeed stress the posterior medial meniscal horns, it is wise to restrict flexion to no greater than 90° for the first 4 weeks. After 6 weeks of toe-touch weight-bearing, advancement to full weight-bearing is gradually allowed, and physical therapy is prescribed for further range of motion gains and quadriceps/hamstring strengthening. Light jogging is permissible at approximately 3.5 months, although deep squatting is avoided for 4 months following the repair. Return to impact activities like sports is generally discouraged until 5 months postoperatively.

Results

Clearly, the results of root avulsion repair are directly related to the amount of degenerative changes present. Perhaps the largest series on root repair is by Lee et al. [17]. These investigators report that most of their patients were satisfied with their results. Most impressive is the lack of advancement of degenerative changes seen over a minimum 2-year follow-up. This suggests that restoration of hoop stresses to meniscal tissue may serve as a chondral protective agent.

Following repair, patients appear to enjoy a diminution of pain, which is likely due to the enhanced "cushioning" effect afforded by the now competent meniscus. This is analogous to the pain relief experienced by patients undergoing meniscal transplantation.

Jung et al. described using an all-inside repair with a suture anchor to repair a root tear of the medial meniscus [18]. In their case series, they evaluated clinical and objective outcomes after medial meniscal root repairs in thirteen patients. At an average follow-up of 30.8 months, no patients had joint line tenderness, effusion, catching, or giving way of their knees. The mean Tegner activity level increased from 1.9 ± 1.4 preop to 3.9 ± 1.3 postoperatively. Follow-up MRI showed complete healing in 50% of patients at 6 months post-op.

Kim et al. looked at results of pull-out repairs to treat 30 medial meniscal root tears. In their series, the mean Lysholm score increased to 77.2 postoperatively from 46.2 preoperatively. Postoperative MRI scans showed complete healing in 56.7% of patients and partial healing in 36.7%, however no significant improvement in meniscal extrusion [19]. Seo et al. also used a pull-out repair in 21 medial meniscal root tears [20]. Their series also showed an increase in mean Lysholm score to 83.0 postoperatively from 56.1 preoperatively. Eleven patients in this series had second-look arthroscopy which showed scar healing in 36.4%, lax healing in 45.5%, and no healing in 18.2%.

While further long-term follow-up studies examining the results of meniscal root repair as well as further studies evaluating the optimal repair techniques are needed, these early studies looking at results suggest that appreciable symptomatic relief may be attained, and meniscal root repair indeed appears warranted in properly chosen patients.

Complications

Chondral injury may result from drill guide placement, although there is no available literature regarding the prevalence of this occurrence. Inadvertent drill placement may result in neurovascular injury; however, careful exposure of the horn insertion should help avert this complication. Stiffness may ensue from the prolonged protective weight-bearing; patellar mobilization and early passive ROM may help minimize the occurrence of arthrofibrosis. Use of suture anchors puts patients at risk for anchor loosening necessitating further surgery for anchor removal [18].

Failure to heal may result from several causes. Early weight-bearing will strain the repair and will potentiate gap formation at the meniscal insertion site. Overly aggressive rehabilitation, whereupon early extreme flexion is instituted, will load the repair inordinately and deter healing. Lastly, overly ambitious surgery where tissue quality is indeed poor and chondral injury severe will surely compromise surgical success. During attempts at suture passage, tissue quality must be honestly assessed. Flimsy and fragmented posterior horn tissue cannot be expected to reliably support suture fixation.

Summary

Meniscal root avulsion must be suspected in the setting of patients with joint line pain who do not manifest classic linear signal changes on MR. The presence of meniscal extrusion coupled with separation at the tibial insertion seen on axial cuts supports the diagnosis. The old paradigm of dismissing extruded menisci as merely "arthritis" is no longer tenable. Patients may be afforded appreciable relief of symptoms and perhaps considerable chondral protection from repair of root avulsion.

References

1. Greis PE, Bardana DD, Holmstrom MC, Burks RT. Meniscal injury: I. Basic science and evaluation. J Am Acad Orthop Surg. 2002;10:168–76.
2. Marzo JM. Medial meniscus posterior horn avulsion. J Am Acad Orthop Surg. 2009;17:276–83.
3. Bhattacharyya T, Gale D, Dewire P, et al. The clinical importance of meniscal tears demonstrated by MRI in osteoarthritis of the knee. J Bone Joint Surg Am. 2003;85:4–9.
4. Bin SI, Kim JM, Shin SJ. Radial tears of the posterior horn of the medial meniscus. Arthroscopy. 2004;20: 373–8.
5. Ozkoc G, Circi E, Gonc U, et al. Radial tears in the root if the posterior horn of the medial meniscus. Knee Surg Sports Traumatol Arthrosc. 2008;16:849–54.
6. Allaire R, Muriuki M, Gilbertson L, Harner CD. Mechanical consequences of a tear of the posterior root of the medial meniscus. J Bone Joint Surg Am. 2008;90:1922–31.
7. Marzo JM, Gurske-DePerio J. Effects of medial meniscus posterior horn avulsion and repair on tibiofemoral contact area and peak contact pressure with clinical implications. Am J Sports Med. 2009;37: 124–9.
8. Hein CN, Deperio JG, Ehrensberger MT, Marzo JM. Effects of medial meniscal posterior horn avulsion and repair on meniscal displacement. Knee. 2011;18: 189–92.
9. Berthiaume MJ, Raynauld JP, Martel-Pelletie J, Labonte F, et al. Meniscal tear and extrusion are strongly associated with progression of symptomatic knee osteoarthritis as assessed by quantitative magnetic resonance imaging. Ann Rheum Dis. 2005; 64:556–63.
10. Felson D. An update on the pathogenesis and epidemiology of OA. Radiol Clin North Am. 2004;42:1–9.
11. Hunter DJ. Osteoarthritis. Best Pract Res Clin Rheumatol. 2011;25:801.
12. Hwang BY et al. Risk factors for medial meniscal posterior root tear. Am J Sports Med. 2012;40: 1606–10.
13. Ahmed A et al. In vitro measurement of static pressure distribution in synovial joints—part 1, tibial surface of the knee. J Biomech Eng. 1983;105:216–25.
14. Shelbourne KD, Heinrich J. The long-term evaluation of lateral meniscus tears left in situ at the time of anterior cruciate ligament reconstruction. Arthroscopy. 2004;20:346–51.
15. Harner CD, Mauro CS, Lesniak BP, Romanowski JR. Biomechanical consequences of a tear of the posterior root of the medial meniscus: surgical technique. J Bone Joint Surg Am. 2009;91A:257–70.
16. Kim SJ, Song HT, Moon HK, Chun YM, Chang WH. The safe establishment of a transseptal portal in the posterior knee. Knee Surg Sports Traumatol Arthrosc. 2011;19:1320–5.
17. Lee JH, Lim YJ, Kim KB, Kim KH, Song JH. Arthroscopic pullout repair of posterior root tear of the medial meniscus: radiographic and clinical results with a 2 yr follow up. Arthroscopy. 2009;25:951–8.
18. Jung YH, Choi NH, Oh JS, Victoroff BN. All-inside repair for a root tear of the medial meniscus using a suture anchor. Am J Sports Med. 2012;40:1406–11.
19. Kim SB, Ha JK, Lee SW, et al. Medial meniscus root tear refixation: comparison of clinical, radiologic, and arthroscopic findings with medial meniscectomy. Arthroscopy. 2011;27:346–54.
20. Seo HS, Lee SC, Jung KA. Second-look arthroscopic findings after repair of posterior root tears of the medial meniscus. Am J Sports Med. 2011;39: 99–107.

Indications for Meniscus Repair

9

Scott E. Urch, John D. Kelly IV,
and K. Donald Shelbourne

Abbreviations

ACL   Anterior cruciate ligament
MRI   Magnetic resonance imaging
ROM   Range of motion

Introduction

There has been much recent discussion with the increase in popularity of arthroscopy as to the indications for meniscus repair. The commonly held belief is that without the meniscus, the knee is prone to early osteoarthritis and that preserving the meniscus through meniscal repair will help stop or delay this process. However, not all situations where the meniscus is torn warrant a repair. It is very important to understand what causes a meniscus to tear, what factors affect its ability to heal, and whether a repaired meniscus will function normally or at least provide better function than if the meniscus is removed.

It is also important to distinguish between isolated meniscus tears and those that occur

S.E. Urch, M.D. (✉) • K.D. Shelbourne, M.D.
Shelbourne Knee Center, 1815 N. Capitol Ave.
Suite 600, Indianapolis, IN 46202, USA
e-mail: surch@fixknee.com

J.D. Kelly IV, M.D.
Department of Orthopaedic Surgery, Hospital of the
University of Pennsylvania, 3400 Spruce Street,
2 Silverstein, Philadelphia, PA 19104, USA

concomitant with an anterior cruciate ligament (ACL) tear. In the ACL-intact knee, meniscus tears are usually the result of degenerative changes causing the meniscus to fail. There is usually less energy imparted to cause the meniscal tissue to tear. In the ACL-deficient knee or at the time of an acute ACL injury, excessive joint movement causes a usually structurally sound meniscus to tear as it becomes caught between the tibia and the femur. However, in both acute ACL injuries and in chronically unstable knees, the meniscus may also have a degenerative component. The condition of the meniscus should be a major consideration in the decision of whether or not to proceed with a repair.

The location of the tear and type of tear pattern are other factors that influence the healing potential of a meniscus repair. The blood supply to the meniscus is supplied peripherally by the perimeniscal capillary plexus which extends into 20–30 % of the medial meniscus and 10–25 % of the lateral meniscus [1, 2]. Therefore, the closer the tear is to the periphery of the meniscus, the greater the blood supply that is available to promote healing.

Although they share many qualities, the medial and lateral menisci are quite different in how they function, how they are injured, and how they respond to repair. In general, the lateral meniscus is much more mobile than the medial meniscus. The lateral meniscus has been shown to translate 9–11 mm in the anterior–posterior plane, whereas the medial meniscus has been shown to only have 2–5 mm of translation in the same plane [3]. Most of the posterior capsular attachment of the lateral meniscus is anterior to the popliteus tendon, making the posterior portion more mobile. In contrast, the medial meniscus has a very solid capsular attachment throughout and, therefore, is more rigidly affixed to the tibia. Secondary to its increased translation, the lateral meniscus is more likely to be injured acutely at the time of anterior cruciate ligament injury. In a study of 448 patients with acute ACL injuries, Shelbourne and Gray found that 62 % of patients had lateral meniscus tears and 42 % had medial meniscus tears [4].

By contrast, medial meniscus injuries are more common in conjunction with chronic ACL injuries. In a study of 552 patients with chronic ACL-deficient knees, Cipolla et al. [5] showed a 74 % incidence of medial meniscus tears compared to a 42 % incidence of lateral meniscus tears.

It is believed that a medial meniscus lesion was created at the time of the injury and continued to propagate with additional "pivoting" episodes prior to surgery. Another explanation is that since the posterior horn of the medial meniscus serves as a secondary stabilizer to anterior tibial translation, it realizes increased stress in the presence of ACL insufficiency and finally succumbs to structural failure.

There are also common tear patterns that are peculiar to various injuries, each holding prognostic significance for reparability. For instance, there are two types of lateral meniscus tears associated with an ACL tear injury: (1) a vertical longitudinal tear in the posterior third which may (Fig. 9.1) or may not (Fig. 9.2) extend past the popliteus or (2) an avulsion of the posterior attachment of the meniscus (Fig. 9.3) [6]. Both of these tears are inherently stable and will often

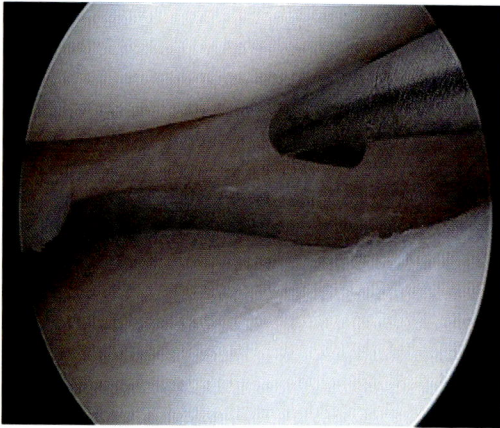

Fig. 9.1 Arthroscopic picture showing a stable, vertical longitudinal tear in the posterior third of the lateral meniscus which does not extend anterior to the popliteal tendon

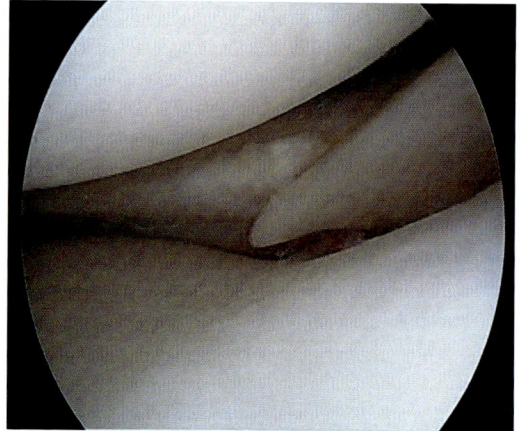

Fig. 9.3 An avulsion of the posterior attachment of the lateral meniscus

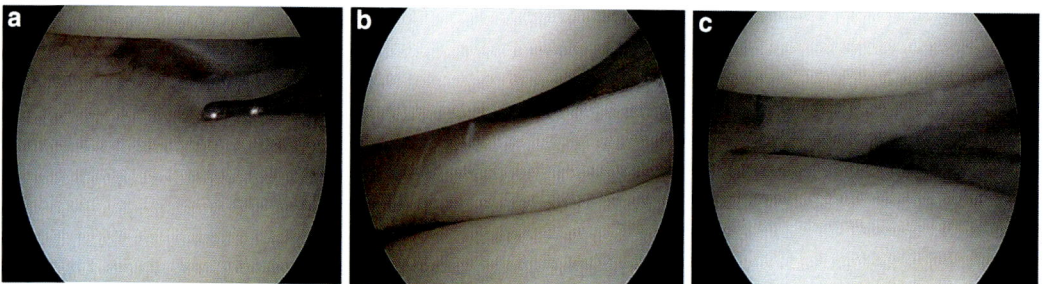

Fig. 9.2 A vertical longitudinal tear of the lateral meniscus that extends anterior to the popliteus (**a**) and can be displaced into the intercondylar notch with a probe (**b**). The same meniscus tear is shown after suture repair (**c**)

times show evidence of healing at the time of the subsequent ACL surgery. Tears along the periphery of the meniscus (red–red or red–white zones) may become unstable the larger they become and can ultimately allow the meniscus to displace if a critical size is reached. When these tears are encountered in conjunction with an acute ACL tear, their size and mobility will dictate if they need to be repaired. However, when these tears have a degenerative component, or they are torn in multiple planes, repair is likely not indicated.

The medial meniscus also has varying tear patterns that are encountered in unique situations, and medial meniscus tears account for the preponderance of arthroscopies done in the United States. The medial meniscus tears that occur at the time of an ACL injury are very similar to those that occur on the lateral side. They tend to be vertical tears in the posterior third which occur when the tibia and the femur are forcefully compressed the time of the index "pivot" episode. These are usually stable tears and, therefore, may be regarded as somewhat incidental findings at the time of ACL reconstruction. In chronic ACL tears, when the knee is subjected to repeated episodes of instability, medial tears can become larger, rendering them unstable tears that are displaceable into the intracondylar notch [7]. In ACL-intact knees, the pattern of tear is distinctly different. These tears are usually degenerative and will predictably tear in both the vertical and horizontal planes, making repair less likely to succeed.

In this chapter we will discuss the general indications for repair of both the medial and lateral menisci in both the ACL-intact knee and in the ACL-injured knee. It is our hope to guide the reader in making more sound and scientifically based decisions in meniscal tear management.

ACL-Intact Knee

Medial Meniscus Tears in the ACL-Intact Knee

It has been estimated that over 850,000 knee arthroscopies are performed annually in the United States for treatment of meniscus tears [8].

Medial meniscus tears are much more common than lateral meniscus tears, and males are more commonly affected at a rate of approximately 2.5:1 [8]. Degenerative tears are most commonly seen in patients over the age of 40, but they can also be seen in younger patients with a history of sports activities involving repeated deep knee flexion, such as wresting, baseball/softball catching, and volleyball. With time and repetitive motion, the meniscus begins to fail usually first in the horizontal plane. This enables the inferior lamina to displace into the joint, allowing it to become compressed between the tibia and the femur. As the "horizontal cleavage" enlarges, it is prone to catch even more, causing increased symptoms and propagation of the tear (Fig. 9.4). Patients often report pain with squatting and rotation, as these activities cause the meniscus to get caught. These tears usually have an insidious onset of swelling, pain, and catching, and they are not usually attributed to a specific injury.

Several studies have shown higher success rates of medial meniscus repairs that were done at the time of ACL reconstruction compared with repairs done in ACL-intact knees [9–12]. Cannon and Vittori [11] evaluated meniscal healing in 90 repairs done in conjunction with ACL reconstruction and 27 repairs done in ACL-intact knees. They concluded that overall, the success was higher when the repair was done in conjunction with ACL reconstruction (93 %) compared to repairs done in an ACL-intact knee (50 %). It has long been assumed that this success is secondary to the bleeding and growth factors associated with an ACL reconstruction. However, as noted earlier, most tears occurring in ACL-injured knees are sustained to a *normal* meniscus, whereas tears in an ACL-intact knee are more often degenerative in nature. Without the presence of good quality meniscal tissue to facilitate healing of the repair, a significantly higher failure rate is to be expected.

A distinct type of tear occurs in the posterior third of the medial meniscus and is seen in patients with early degenerative joint disease. These "root avulsion" or posterior horn detachments are especially common in middle-aged females and are discussed elsewhere (Chap. 12)

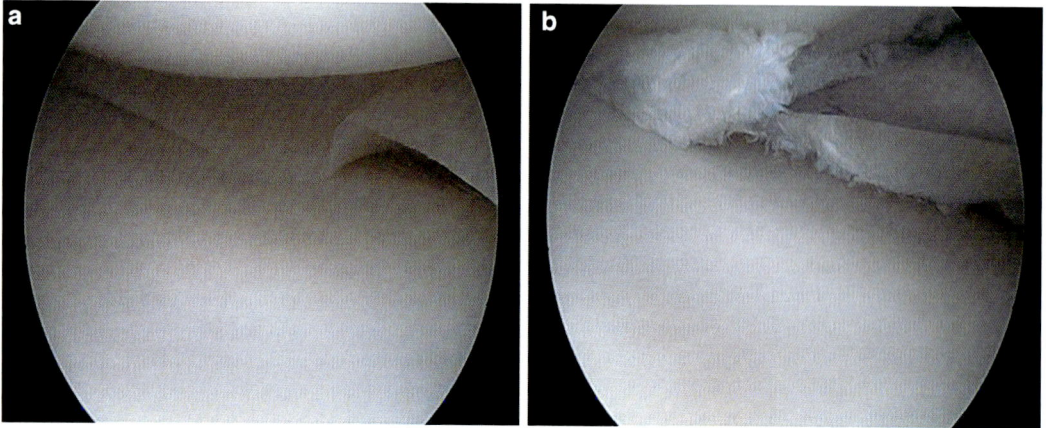

Fig. 9.4 This medial meniscus appears to be normal (**a**) prior to placing the probe into the undersurface of the meniscus where the degenerative tear is located. (**b**) Probing the medial meniscus reveals a vertical tear with a horizontal degenerative component

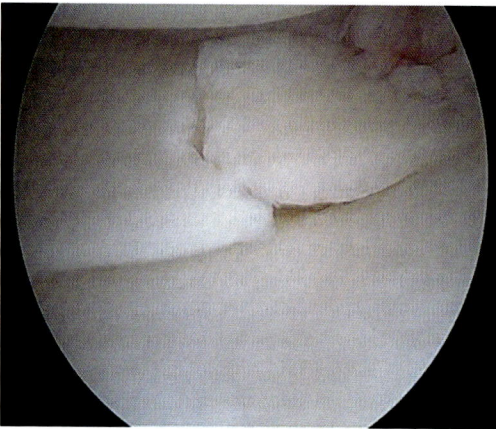

Fig. 9.5 A posterior radial tear of the medial meniscus

in more detail. Unlike lateral posterior horn tears seen in the setting of acute ACL injury, the medial root avulsion tears have a low propensity for spontaneous healing. Patients commonly complain of a specific injury where they felt a distinct tear or pop, usually when stepping up/down a stair or planting the foot. These tears occur near the posterior horn attachment to the tibia (Fig. 9.5), and they are believed to occur as a result of increasing medial side joint stress secondary to chondral wear and decreasing joint space width. Laboratory studies have shown that when these tears are created in a cadaver and then repaired, they will restore normal joint contact

pressures [13, 14]. However, no studies have conclusively shown that repairing these tears can *reverse* the natural course of joint wear and arthritis when the knee already has degenerative changes visible on radiographs. Lee et al. [15] showed that degenerative tears with a radial component showed more evidence of meniscal extrusion than degenerative tears without a radial component. They also found that the presence of a radial component and the severity of osteoarthritis were predictive of extrusion. They recommended that arthroscopic procedures, particularly meniscus repair, should be cautiously considered in cases of meniscal extrusion [15]. A great number of magnetic resonance imaging (MRI) scans done on patients with radiographic evidence of arthritis of the knee will show this type of tear with the meniscus extruded from the joint. In the presence of moderate to severe degenerative changes, repair of this meniscus tear is not likely to result in elimination of symptoms since patient discomfort is primarily due to the arthritic changes. Lim et al. [16] showed in 2010 that these tears can be treated nonoperatively with a decrease in symptoms, lending credence to the idea that the symptoms these patients experience are at least in part related to the osteoarthritis and not the meniscus tear.

However, when Lee et al. [17] examined results of fixation of posterior root tears via a pullout suture technique, they noted that most of their patients were satisfied with their results, showing significant improvement in Hospital for Special Surgery and Lysholm subjective scores. Most impressive is the lack of advancement of degenerative changes seen over a mean follow-up of 31.8 months [17]. Although longer-term follow-up is warranted, this suggests that restoration of hoop stresses to meniscal tissue may serve as a chondral protective agent.

Lateral Meniscus Tears in the ACL-Intact Knee

As mentioned previously, the lateral meniscus has a very different tibial anchoring mechanism than the medial side; specifically, it does not have a significant attachment to the posterior third of the capsule and, subsequently, is more mobile. This increased mobility can predispose the lateral meniscus to result in a displaced bucket-handle tear when more violent torsional stress is applied. Increased forward mobility of the meniscus can predispose to a tissue failure, particularly anterior to the popliteus tendon, and propagation until the meniscus gets "wedged" within the intercondylar notch. This differs from what occurs on the medial side where a bucket-handle medial meniscus tear will usually flip 180° from its normal position when it displaces; the lateral meniscus will simply slide into the notch in its normal planar orientation. Clinically, patients with these tears often present reporting pain after rising quickly from a position with their legs crossed or with their knees in a figure-4 position. Most often, these tears are nondegenerative and, therefore, are amenable to repair (Fig. 9.2). Since the attachment to the capsule is anterior to the popliteus tendon, that is the portion of the tear that needs most attention during repair. The authors prefer an inside-out suture technique, but any system or "fixator" that allows the meniscus to be secured both superiorly and inferiorly will suffice.

The other acute tear pattern commonly seen in the lateral meniscus is a radial tear (Fig. 9.6). These tears are most often seen in the mid-third of the meniscus and are associated with a valgus

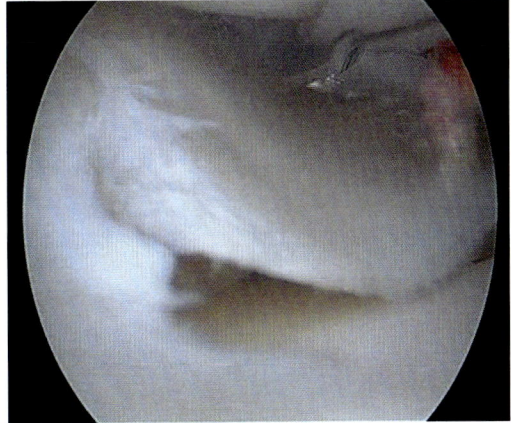

Fig. 9.6 A radial tear of the lateral meniscus

injury or a valgus rotational injury. As the joint opens medially during valgus loading, the lateral meniscus is compressed and tears in a radial fashion. The fibers of the meniscus are oriented in a parallel and circular pattern creating a hoop. Radial tears disrupt this hoop force and render the meniscus much less effective in dissipating stress. Radial tears of the lateral meniscus are commonly in the white–white zone and, consequently, are usually not amenable to repair. There have been studies advocating for repair of these tears, especially when biologic augmentation is employed. However, it is the authors' practice to remove the torn portion back to stable fibers in order to prevent tear propagation.

Although relatively uncommon, the meniscus can be developmentally formed aberrantly in the form of a discoid meniscus. These flat, pancake-resembling structures are seen more frequently in Asian populations and are often structurally unsound. Furthermore, a discoid meniscus may tear because its abnormal shape renders it unable to sustain more joint compression. A discoid lateral meniscus is far more common than a discoid medial meniscus. The discoid tear frequently occurs in the structurally abnormal area of the meniscus found directly under the femoral condyle. Consequently, it is not amenable to repair. Instead, it is removed back to the portion of the meniscus which is normal. However, the Wrisberg variant, or detachment of the posterior horn from the posterior capsule, is amenable to repair.

Great care must be taken during suturing of these lesions as the posterior horn of the lateral meniscus is directly anterior to the popliteal artery. For inside-out techniques, a contralateral suturing portal must be employed.

Although much less common than degenerative medial meniscus tears, degenerative lateral meniscus tears can occur as well. As with degenerative tears of the medial meniscus, degenerative lateral meniscus tears occur because of attritional changes of the meniscus rather than because of an acute injury. They are often seen in conjunction with degenerative changes in the lateral compartment, and just like on the medial side, the lateral meniscus can be extruded when joint space narrowing is present. Of course, attempts to repair this type of meniscus tear are usually doomed to fail because of the poor quality of the meniscus.

ACL-Deficient Knee

Much research in the last several years has focused on the treatment of meniscus tears that occur with ACL injury. We have known for many years that if the ACL is left untreated, there is a much higher risk of meniscus injury, particularly to the medial meniscus [7]. As a result, there has been increased awareness of the types of injuries that occur with ACL tears and how they should be treated.

Lateral Meniscus Tears in the ACL-Deficient Knee

As stated, several studies have shown that the lateral meniscus is more commonly torn acutely at the time of ACL injury [4, 5]. This is likely because the meniscus becomes trapped between the femur and the tibia during the acute pivoting episode. Most commonly, the tear occurs in the posterior third of the lateral meniscus, which does not have a strong attachment to the surrounding capsule. However, the indications for repair of this lesion are bathed in controversy. In their study of 178 lateral meniscus tears left in situ at the time of ACL reconstruction, Fitzgibbons and Shelbourne [6] found that 52 were posterior horn avulsions, 99 were stable vertical tears of the posterior horn, and 27 were stable non-displaced vertical tears that extended anterior to the popliteus. Several studies have shown that these meniscus tears can be left in situ without risk of retear or further significant injury [6, 18–20]. Often times, the authors will trephinate the portion that is torn if it does not appear to be completely healed at the time of surgery. Trephination has been shown in both animal and clinical studies to promote meniscal healing by creating vascular channels [11, 21, 22]. Since these longitudinal tears are generally stable, there is no need for formal fixation, but stimulation of the surrounding tissue helps promote healing. Shelbourne and Heinrich reported on 43 patients who had trephination of posterior or peripheral lateral meniscus tears at the time of ACL reconstruction and found that none required any additional surgery at a mean follow-up of 6.6 years postoperatively [20].

Occasionally the lateral meniscus tear can extend anterior to the popliteus, allowing the fragment to displace. When this occurs on the medial side, the knee will become "stuck" preventing full extension; however, on the lateral side, the knee does not get locked when the meniscus displaces into the intercondylar notch because it occupies the portion of the notch where the ACL would normally be located. These patients may be able to obtain full range of motion (ROM) despite the displacement of the large fragment of the meniscus. If this tear is not degenerative, then a repair should be considered. Again, we use an inside-out suture repair which has a low risk of chondral damage or migration and, subsequently, a low rate of complications.

Finally, Shelbourne et al. [23] have noted strong evidence of healing of lateral meniscal root avulsions left in situ at the time of ACL reconstruction (Fig. 9.3). In a group of 33 patients with a mean objective follow-up of 10.6 years, no reoperations were required for removal of the meniscus tear, subjective scores were not statistically significantly different than the control group, and only mild joint space narrowing (1 ± 1.6 mm) was found [23]. Thus, it is our belief that these tears can be left "in situ," although this remains controversial.

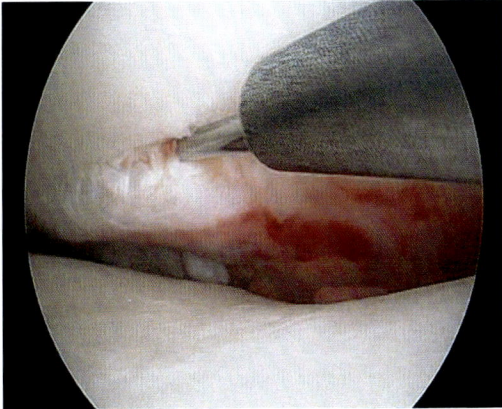

Fig. 9.7 Stable vertical medial meniscus tear being trephinated to stimulate vascular flow into the tear

Medial Meniscus Tears in the ACL-Deficient Knee

On the medial side, the meniscus tears that occur in conjunction with ACL tears are somewhat similar to what is seen on the medial side in an ACL-intact knee. The most common type of medial meniscus tear seen with acute ACL injury is a vertical tear in the peripheral vascular zone, generally at the junction of the posterior and middle third. It is caused by compression of the femur on the tibia at the time of the acute pivoting episode. These tears are seen at the time of ACL surgery, but they can also be detected on preoperative MRI if one is obtained. Many of these tears are fairly small (<1 cm) and are stable when probed. When this is the case, there is some evidence that they can be trephinated to stimulate vascular inflow into the tear (Fig. 9.7), with formal repair not necessary when the ACL is reconstructed at the same time. Shelbourne and Rask [24] showed that if the tear could not be displaced into the joint, even tears longer than 1 cm showed good results with trephination. Between 1982 and 1988, 139 stable tears were left in situ. Between 1989 and 1997, 233 stable tears were treated with abrasion and trephination. At a mean of 3.7 years after surgery, a subsequent arthroscopy for meniscus tear was required for only 15 of the 139 tears left in situ (10.8 %) and 14 of the 233 tears that were trephinated (6 %) [24].

It is very important to thoroughly probe the tear, looking for a secondary horizontal cleavage component (Fig. 9.4). The presence of horizontal extension indicates that the tear has a degenerative component, making meniscectomy more reasonable than meniscal repair or trephination.

Several studies have shown that meniscus tears repaired at the time of ACL reconstruction have good healing potential [9, 11, 25–27]. Although all of these tears *can* heal, several factors were identified to help determine more precisely the likelihood of a meniscus tear to heal:

- Tears that are smaller and closer to the periphery seem to have the best results.
- Tears that are large, displaced, or/and complex are less likely and/or heal.
- Tears that are located in the central-third area, which is less vascular, are less likely to heal.

In general, tears that occur acutely with an ACL tear will occur more in the peripheral region of the meniscus, but as the tear becomes more degenerative, the tear location is found more in the central portion of the meniscus. Although these tears *can* heal, the question really is do they function as they should to protect the joint, and do they cause symptoms for the patient in the future?

Shelbourne and Carr [28] compared the results of meniscus repair versus partial meniscectomy of bucket-handle medial meniscus tears in ACL-reconstructed patients. None of the patients had lateral meniscus tears or chondral damage greater than Outerbridge Grade 2. The expectation was that patients with meniscal repair would fare better symptomatically than those with meniscectomy. At a mean follow-up of 8 years after surgery, there was no difference between groups, with both groups having a mean modified Noyes score of 90.9 [28]. When the repair group was analyzed based on whether the bucket-handle tear was degenerative or nondegenerative, the mean score for patients with repaired degenerative tears was significantly lower than the mean score for patients with repaired nondegenerative tears, 87.1 and 93.9, respectively [28]. It is interesting to note that in a recent paper, Shelbourne and Gray [29] presented 10–15-year follow-up on 502 patients with ACL reconstruction. They found that patients who had no meniscus pathology at the time of

Modified Noyes Scores
Based on ROM and Meniscal Status

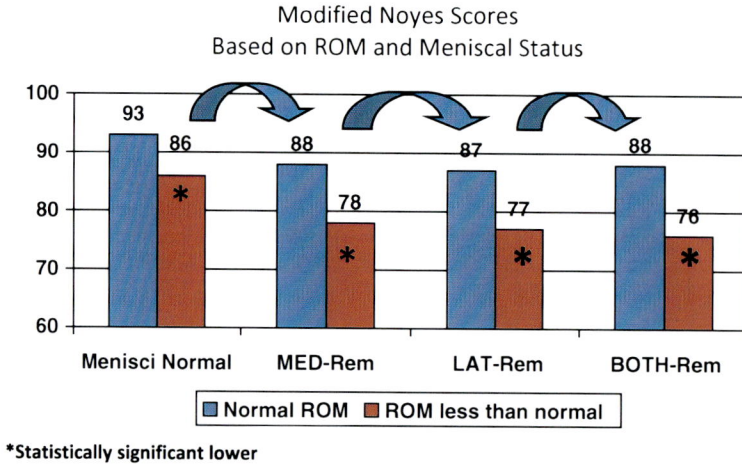

*Statistically significant lower

Fig. 9.8 Modified Noyes scores based on range of motion (ROM) status at 10–20-year follow-up for patients with normal menisci and patients who underwent meniscectomy. Despite having a meniscectomy, patients who were able to maintain normal ROM had similar scores to patients with normal menisci. Lower subjective scores were observed in all groups when full ROM was not maintained

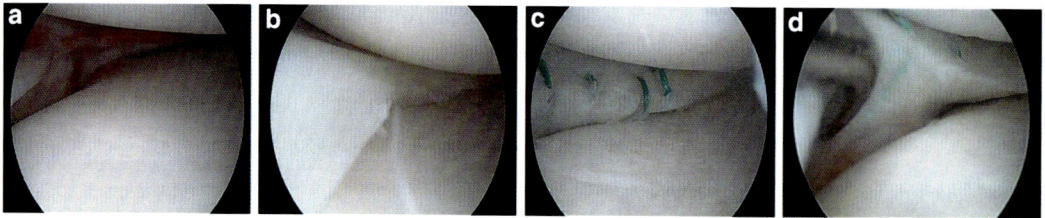

Fig. 9.9 (**a**) A bucket-handle medial meniscus tear displaced into the intercondylar notch. (**b**) A bucket-handle medial meniscus tear after being reduced. (**c**) Immediately after suture repair of a bucket-handle medial meniscus tear. (**d**) Second-look arthroscopy 6 weeks after suture repair of a bucket-handle medial meniscus tear

their ACL reconstruction and maintained full ROM in their knee rated their knee at 93, whereas those that had a medial meniscectomy at the time of their ACL reconstruction rated their knee at 88 (Fig. 9.8) [29]. Indeed, loss of meniscal tissue translates to increased morbidity. However, the repair study suggests that although the meniscus may heal, if it is a degenerative tear, it may not provide any additional function than what would be provided by the remaining meniscus after a partial meniscectomy, especially if full ROM is maintained [28, 29]. In an effort to prevent degenerative changes in the knee, the current mantra seems to be an "attempt to preserve the meniscus at all cost." However, there is a high rate of reoperation in patients with meniscal repairs, suggesting that a better understanding of the mechanics of the meniscus function and healing potential of different tear patterns is warranted before meniscus repair is recommended.

When the tear is very large, it may become unstable and displace into the intercondylar notch, a "bucket-handle" tear (Fig. 9.9a). Patients will occasionally present with this at the time of ACL injury, but this is much more common with chronic ACL tears. If a patient cannot completely straighten their knee, and they do not respond to rehabilitation exercises to improve knee extension, then an MRI scan is indicated to determine if the meniscus is displaced into the intercondylar notch, blocking extension. The younger the age of the patient, the lower the chance that the tear would have a degenerative component, making meniscus repair more likely. In these cases, arthroscopy is needed to reduce the meniscus from the notch in order to allow for full knee extension prior to proceeding with the ACL reconstruction (Fig. 9.9b–d). There is a much higher risk of arthrofibrosis in patients who do not have normal ROM prior to ACL reconstruction [30]. Therefore, the authors suggest considering a "staged approach," first performing an arthroscopy to correct and repair the meniscus, then proceeding with ACL reconstruction at a later date once full, symmetric ROM has been achieved. Shelbourne and Johnson [31] found a higher incidence of arthrofibrosis in patients who underwent meniscus repair or removal of a locked bucket-handle meniscus tear in conjunction with ACL reconstruction versus patients who underwent staged procedures of meniscus repair or removal, followed by a period of rehabilitation to restore normal ROM, and finally ACL reconstruction. With increasing age of the patient or longer time intervals between ACL injury and surgery, there is increased likelihood of a degenerative type of tear. Since a meniscectomy may be the best option in this circumstance, if no repairable "bucket-handle" type of tear is present, it may be possible to return ROM prior to surgery and perform a meniscectomy at the time of ACL reconstruction.

Conclusion

Over the years, much research has focused on identifying optimal ways to treat varying types of meniscus tears. Historically, the emphasis has focused on attempting to preserve the meniscus at all costs to help ensure the overall health of the knee. However, in recent years there has been significant evidence indicating that the status of the meniscus is only one of *many* factors influencing the overall long-term health of the knee. It has been shown by Shelbourne and Gray [29] that ROM, particularly knee extension, is the single most important factor in determining how the knee functions long term after ACL reconstruction. The loss of the meniscus, either medial or lateral, was also a significant factor in the regression analysis, but with lower impact than ROM loss (Fig. 9.8) [29]. At 10–20 years after

ACL reconstruction, if both menisci were normal at the time of surgery, the mean Modified Noyes score was 93 if ROM motion was symmetric. However, if ROM was not symmetric, then the mean Modified Noyes score was 86. If the medial, lateral, or both menisci were removed at the time of the initial surgery, and motion was maintained symmetric to the opposite side, then the mean Modified Noyes scores were 88, 87, and 88 for those groups, respectively. If ROM was less than normal, the mean scores dropped by at least 10 points for each group. This suggests that although we should try to preserve the meniscus when possible, removing the meniscus when appropriate is not as consequential to long-term outcomes as loss of motion.

We must always keep in mind the differences between the medial and lateral meniscus. The lateral meniscus is much more mobile and more tolerant to *mild* rotation than the more rigidly affixed medial meniscus. A meniscus should be repaired when it is a nondegenerative tear that has increased instability, such as tears of the lateral side that extend anterior to the popliteus, or in the case of the medial side when there is a vertical tear without a horizontal degenerative component. These should be stabilized to prevent further meniscal excursion and propagation of the tear. We prefer an inside-out suture repair, but whatever method will stabilize the meniscus without further damage to the joint should be considered. Whenever there is a tear to the meniscus that has tissue disruption in more than one plane—representing degeneration—a repair may not be the best course of action.

References

1. Arnoczky SP, Warren RF. Microvasculature of the human meniscus. Am J Sports Med. 1982;10:90–5.
2. Arnoczky SP, Warren RF. The microvasculature of the meniscus and its response to injury: an experimental study in the dog. Am J Sports Med. 1983;11:131–41.
3. Maitra RS, Miller MD, Johnson DL. Meniscal reconstruction. Part I: indications, techniques, and graft considerations. Am J Orthop. 1999;28:213–8.
4. Shelbourne KD, Gray T. Anterior cruciate ligament reconstruction with autogenous patellar tendon graft

followed by accelerated rehabilitation: a two- to nine-year followup. Am J Sports Med. 1997;25:786–95.

5. Cipolla M, Scala A, Gianni E, Puddu G. Different patterns of meniscal tears in acute anterior ligament (ACL) ruptures and in chronic ACL-deficient knees. Knee Surg Sports Traumatol Arthrosc. 1995;3:130–4.

6. Fitzgibbons RE, Shelbourne KD. "Aggressive" nontreatment of lateral meniscal tears seen during anterior cruciate ligament reconstruction. Am J Sports Med. 1995;23:156–9.

7. Yoo JC, Ahn JH, Lee SH, Yoon YC. Increasing incidence of medial meniscus tears in nonoperatively treated anterior cruciate ligament insufficiency patients documented by serial magnetic resonance imaging studies. Am J Sports Med. 2009;8:1478–83.

8. Arendt EA, editor. Orthopaedic knowledge update: sports medicine 2. Rosemont, IL: American Academy of Orthopaedic Surgeons; 1999.

9. Krych AJ, Pitts RT, Dajani KA, Stuart MJ, Levy BA, Dahm DL. Surgical repair of medial meniscus tears with concomitant anterior cruciate ligament reconstruction in patients 18 years and younger. Am J Sports Med. 2010;38(5):976–82.

10. Kurzweil PR, Tifford CD, Ignacio EM. Unsatisfactory clinical results of meniscal repair using the meniscus arrow. Arthroscopy. 2005;21(8):905.e1–7.

11. Cannon Jr WD, Vittori JM. The incidence of healing in arthroscopic meniscal repairs in anterior cruciate ligament-reconstructed knees versus stable knees. Am J Sports Med. 1992;20:176–81.

12. Noyes FR, Barber-Westin SD. Arthroscopic repair of meniscus tears extending into the avascular zone with or without anterior cruciate ligament reconstruction in patients 40 years of age and older. Arthroscopy. 2000;16:822–9.

13. Harner CD, Mauro CS, Lesniak BP, Romanowski JR. Biomechanical consequences of a tear of the posterior root of the medial meniscus. Surgical technique. J Bone Joint Surg Am. 2008;91 Suppl 2:257–70.

14. Marzo JM, Guerske-DePerio J. Effects of medial meniscus posterior horn avulsion and repair on tibiofemoral contact area and peak contact pressure with clinical implications. Am J Sports Med. 2009;37(1):124–9.

15. Lee DH, Lee BS, Kim JM, et al. Predictors of degenerative medial meniscus extrusion, radial component and knee osteoarthritis. Knee Surg Sports Traumatol Arthrosc. 2011;19(2):222–9.

16. Lim HC, Bae JH, Wang JH, Seok CW, Kim MK. Nonoperative treatment of degenerative posterior root tear of the medial meniscus. Knee Surg Sports Traumatol Arthrosc. 2010;18:535–9.

17. Lee JH, Lim YJ, Kim KB, Kim KH, Song JH. Arthroscopic pullout repair of posterior root tear of the medial meniscus: radiographic and clinical results with a 2 yr follow up. Arthroscopy. 2009;25:951–8.

18. Talley MC, Grana WA. Treatment of partial meniscal tears identified during anterior cruciate ligament reconstruction with limited synovial abrasion. Arthroscopy. 2000;16:6–10.

19. Yagashita K, Muneta T, Ogiuchi T, Sekiya I, Shinomiya K. Healing potential of meniscal tears without repair in knees with anterior cruciate ligament reconstruction. Am J Sports Med. 2004;32:1953–61.

20. Shelbourne KD, Heinrich J. The long term evaluation of lateral meniscus tears left in situ at the time of anterior cruciate ligament reconstruction. Arthroscopy. 2004;20:346–51.

21. Zhang Z, Arnold JA, Williams T, McCann B. Repairs by trephination and suturing of longitudinal injuries in the avascular area of the meniscus in goats. Am J Sports Med. 1995;23:35–41.

22. Zhang ZN, Tu KY, Xu YK, Zhang WM, Liu ZT, Ou SH. Treatment of longitudinal injuries in the avascular area of meniscus in dogs by trephination. Arthroscopy. 1988;4:151–9.

23. Shelbourne KD, Roberson TA, Gray T. Long-term evaluation of posterior lateral meniscus root tears left in situ at the time of anterior cruciate ligament reconstruction. Am J Sports Med. 2011;39(7):1439–43.

24. Shelbourne KD, Rask BP. The sequelae of salvaged non degenerative peripheral vertical medial meniscus tears with anterior cruciate ligament reconstruction. Arthroscopy. 2001;17:270–4.

25. Asahina S, Muneta T, Yamamoto H. Arthroscopic meniscal repair in conjunction with anterior cruciate ligament reconstruction: factors affecting the healing rate. Arthroscopy. 1996;12:541–5.

26. O'Shea JJ, Shelbourne KD. Repair of locked bucket handle meniscal tears with chronic anterior cruciate ligament deficiency. Am J Sports Med. 2003;31:216–20.

27. Rubman MH, Noyes FR, Barber-Westin SD. Arthroscopic repair of meniscus tears that extend into the avascular zone: a review of 198 single and complex tears. Am J Sports Med. 1998;26:87–95.

28. Shelbourne KD, Carr DR. Meniscal repair compared with meniscectomy for bucket-handle medial meniscus tears in anterior cruciate ligament reconstructed knees. Am J Sports Med. 2003;31:718–23.

29. Shelbourne KD, Gray T. Minimum 10-year results after anterior cruciate ligament reconstruction: how the loss of normal knee motion compounds other factors related to the development of osteoarthritis after surgery. Am J Sports Med. 2009;37:471–80.

30. Shelbourne KD, Wilckens JH, Mollabashy A, DeCarlo M. Arthrofibrosis in acute anterior cruciate ligament reconstruction: the effect of timing of reconstruction and rehabilitation. Am J Sports Med. 1991;19:332–6.

31. Shelbourne KD, Johnson GE. Locked bucket-handle meniscal tears in knees with chronic anterior cruciate ligament deficiency. Am J Sports Med. 1993;21:779–82.

Basic Science of Meniscus Repair: Limitations and Emerging Strategies

10

Feini Qu, Matthew B. Fisher, and Robert L. Mauck

Abbreviations

ACI	Autologous chondrocyte implantation
bFGF	Basic fibroblast growth factor
CMI	Collagen meniscus implant
ECM	Extracellular matrix
GFP	Green fluorescent protein
IGF-1	Insulin-like growth factor 1
IL-1ra	IL-1 receptor antagonist
IL-1β	Interleukin-1beta
MMP	Matrix metalloproteinase
MSC	Mesenchymal stem cell
PCP	Perimeniscal capillary plexus
PDGF-AB	Platelet-derived growth factor AB
TGF-β	Transforming growth factor beta
TNFα	Tumor necrosis factor alpha
TNFα mAB	Anti-TNFα monoclonal antibody
VEGF	Vascular endothelial growth factor

F. Qu, B.S.E. • M.B. Fisher, Ph.D.
Department of Orthopaedic Surgery, University
of Pennsylvania, 424 Stemmler Hall, 36th Street
and Hamilton Walk, Philadelphia, PA 19104, USA

R.L. Mauck, Ph.D. (✉)
Mckay Orthopaedic Research Laboratory, University
of Pennsylvania, Philadelphia, PA, USA
e-mail: lemauck@mail.med.upenn.edu

Introduction

The meniscus, a semilunar fibrocartilaginous tissue located between the femur and tibia, is essential to the mechanical functionality of the knee. Besides contributing to joint congruency, stability, and shock absorption, it plays a significant role in load bearing, where it transmits the radial components of femoral contact stress into tensile hoop stresses that are resisted at the horns on the tibia [1]. Circumferentially aligned type I collagen fibers, the primary component of the extracellular matrix (ECM), give rise to anisotropic mechanical properties that allow the meniscus to bear greater tensile stresses along the fiber direction [2]. Load-bearing capability decreases when the fiber-reinforced microstructure is compromised, consequently increasing tibiofemoral contact pressures and predisposing the joint to degenerative osteoarthritis (OA). The incidence of meniscal tears is reported to be 60–70 per 100,000 persons [3, 4] and accounts for approximately 850,000 arthroscopic procedures each year [5]. While repair success ranges from 63 % to 91 % for simple peripheral tears [6–11], tears in the inner avascular zone of the meniscus have a much poorer prognosis, with up to 75 % failing to heal completely and 20 % requiring repeat surgery [12]. Partial meniscectomy is the standard treatment after repair failure, yet tissue resection also leads to osteoarthritic changes in the affected knee compartment [13, 14]. Furthermore, it appears that degenerative changes positively correlate with amount of meniscal resection. As such, methods that improve meniscal repair or salvage would be a marked advance to the treatment of this common injury.

This chapter will begin by reviewing the basic science understanding of the limited endogenous healing capacity of the meniscus, with an emphasis on the implications of hypovascularity, hypocellularity, and inflammation at the tear site. Following this discussion, we will describe extant and emerging regenerative medicine approaches that are designed to directly address these issues. This section will include a review of repair strategies and experimental methods that are aimed at (1) enhancing vascularity, (2) increasing cellularity, and (3) promoting matrix deposition and new tissue formation via biochemical and/or mechanical cues at the wound site.

Limitations in Endogenous Meniscus Repair

Multiple factors influence the intrinsic healing capacity of the meniscus, the most significant being zonal differences in vascularity, alterations in matrix composition and density, insufficient cellular density, and other soluble and mechanical factors (Fig. 10.1). Each of these factors is described below as they relate to compromised endogenous healing in the adult meniscus.

Vascular Supply and Meniscus Healing

Healing is characterized by cellular invasion into the defect, with subsequent proliferation, ECM remodeling, and synthesis of new matrix proteins to bridge the wound gap. Thus, the availability of a vascular supply that can deliver regenerative cells, nutrients, and growth factors is likely to be crucial to a successful repair response. The region-specific healing that is seen clinically is largely attributed to degrees of vascularity, where limited vascularization precludes the formation of a fibrin clot that stimulates cellular infiltration and matrix remodeling in the inner, avascular zones of the tissue. Since vessels from the perimeniscal capillary plexus fail to penetrate past the peripheral one-third of the meniscus in the adult (red–red

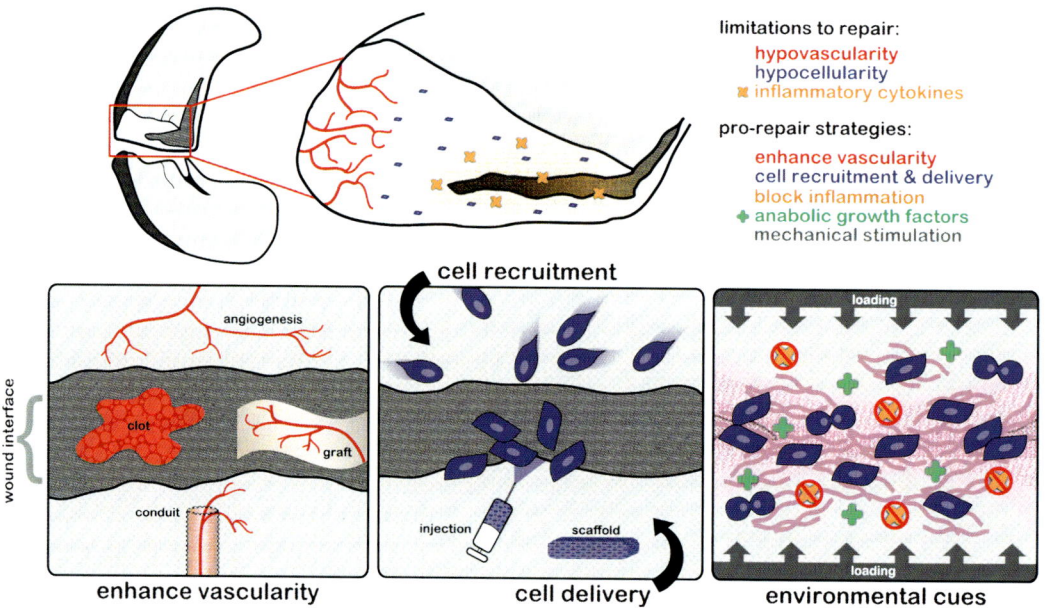

Fig. 10.1 Schematic of a horizontal meniscal tear highlighting the limitations to repair (hypovascularity, hypocellularity, and inflammation) and pro-repair strategies, including enhancing vascularity (angiogenesis, fibrin clot, vascularized graft or conduit), improving cellularity (recruitment or delivery) and generating an instructive environment via biochemical (inflammatory inhibitors and anabolic growth factors) and mechanical cues (dynamic loading)

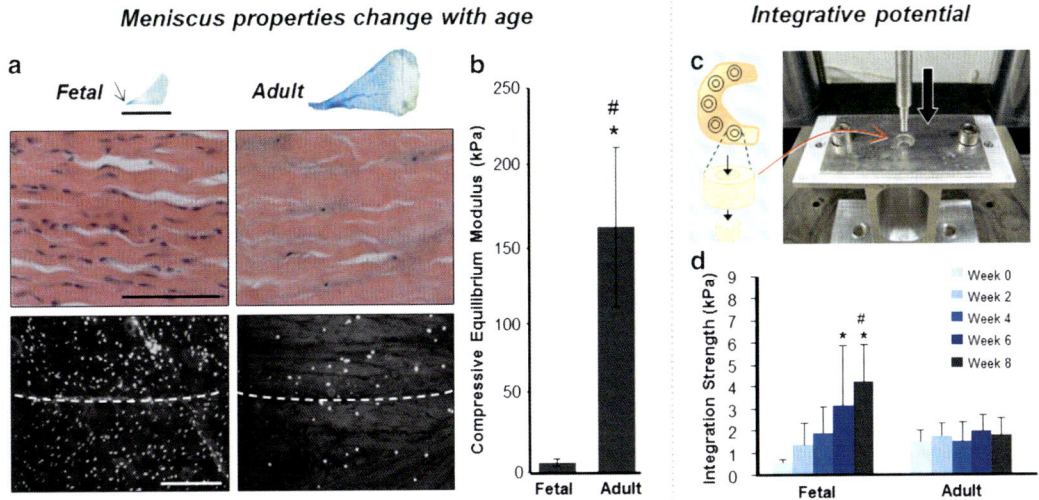

Fig. 10.2 Meniscus properties change with age, contributing to a reduced integrative potential in mature patients. (a) Matrix proteoglycan content and collagen density increase in the adult meniscus (*arrow* indicates the inner zone's concentration of proteoglycans) [24], while cellularity decreases compared to fetal meniscus (*dashed line* indicates wound interface) [127]. (b) The compressive modulus of adult bovine meniscus is greater than that of fetal meniscus [24]. (c) Integration is tested by pushing a cylindrical core out from a surrounding annulus [24]. (d) Integration strength for adult meniscus is lower than fetal meniscus and does not improve with time in culture [24]

zone) [15, 16], this results in an inner avascular zone (white–white zone) with poor healing capacity [17–20]. Junctional tears (red–white zone), as expected, possess intermediate healing capacity. Thus, attempted repair of an avascular tear has a high failure rate and is generally not recommended despite the pathological consequences of partial meniscus removal [21, 22].

Cell and Matrix Density and Meniscus Healing

The presence of a sufficient number of cells at the wound interface is also critical in the healing response. Meniscal cells normally are responsible for maintaining meniscus structure, an active process wherein the ECM is continuously being remodeled due to physiologic loading. These same cells can respond to injury or altered loading by upregulating production of matrix proteins and/or enzymes to affect repair. However, cellularity decreases progressively with maturation until a low cell density is reached in the adult [23, 24] (Fig. 10.2a). Along with a loss in cellularity,

meniscus collagen and proteoglycan content increases with age, increasing the overall ECM density and compressive modulus (Fig. 10.2a, b). The lack of viable cell density in older patients renders them more susceptible to meniscal degeneration and re-tear after repair [25] (Fig. 10.2c, d). Furthermore, the increased ECM density likely reduces the capacity of endogenous cells to migrate and remodel the tissue after injury [23, 24]. In addition to changes that occur with maturation, there are also zonal differences of the cells within the meniscus itself. A superior healing response is often seen in the peripheral region, even after eliminating contributions from the microvasculature and synovium, indicating that there may be intrinsic zonal cellular differences that influence repair [26]. Cell morphology and gene expression vary with meniscal region, with fusiform cells located superficially, fibroblast-like cells in the fibrous periphery, and chondrocyte-like cells in the inner fibrocartilage [27–30]. ECM components also differ by region, where the outer portion consists mainly of type I collagen (80 %) to resist tensile stresses and the inner portion has a greater percentage of type II collagen and proteoglycans, which are more resistant to compressive forces [31] (Fig. 10.2a). As a result, there are zonal differences in regenerative mechanisms, sensitivity to cytokines, and response to growth factors [30].

Thus, introduction of bioactive factors which modulate inflammation and potentiate anabolism and/or loading of the extracellular milieu has the potential to create a matrix-forming environment more conducive to repair.

Soluble and Mechanical Factors and Meniscus Healing

Meniscal healing is also influenced by soluble and mechanical cues. Inflammatory cytokines that are upregulated post-injury, especially interleukin-1beta (IL-1β) and tumor necrosis factor alpha (TNFα), inhibit integrative repair [32]. Specifically, IL-1β increases the expression of matrix metalloproteinases (MMPs), catabolic enzymes that cleave collagens and other ECM components [33]. On the other hand, cells are stimulated to proliferate and produce matrix when exposed to anabolic growth factors. Mechanical loading, such as static or dynamic compression, can also alter gene expression and modulate inflammation [34, 35].

Emerging Strategies to Promote Meniscus Repair

Numerous techniques have been investigated to address the biologic issues of suboptimal meniscus healing and to improve repair (Fig. 10.1). One approach is to enhance vascularity by increasing access to preexisting vasculature or promoting neovascularization to improve delivery of nutrients, reparative cells, and growth factors to the wound site (Fig. 10.3). Another method is to improve the cellularity of the interface by recruiting endogenous cells or introducing exogenous cells (Fig. 10.4). A related approach is to then encourage the cell population to proliferate and increase matrix synthesis by introducing

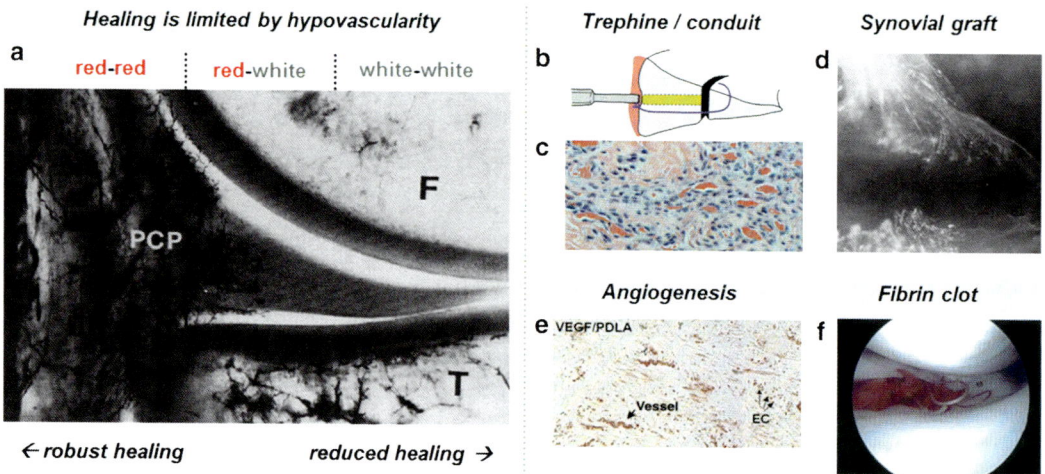

Fig. 10.3 Lack of vasculature in the inner meniscus (white–white zone) results in limited healing after injury. (**a**) Vascular perfusion shows the perimeniscal capillary plexus (PCP) of the medial meniscus (reprinted by permission of SAGE Publications from reference [16]). Strategies to enhance vascularity include increasing vascular access via a trephine/conduit or synovial graft, promoting angiogenesis, and introducing vascular elements. (**b**) Trephine/conduit schematic. (**c**) Tissue and vascular ingrowth using bioabsorbable conduit (reprinted by permission of SAGE Publications from reference [43]). (**d**) Synovial graft placed above meniscal allograft results in vascularization after 8 weeks as seen by microangiography (reprinted with permission from Springer from reference [47]). (**e**) Factor VIII immunostaining indicates early vessel formation in meniscus repaired with VEGF-coated sutures (reprinted with permission from Springer Science and Business Media from reference [50]). (**f**) Fibrin clot placed into meniscal tear with sutures (reprinted with permission from Elsevier from reference [65])

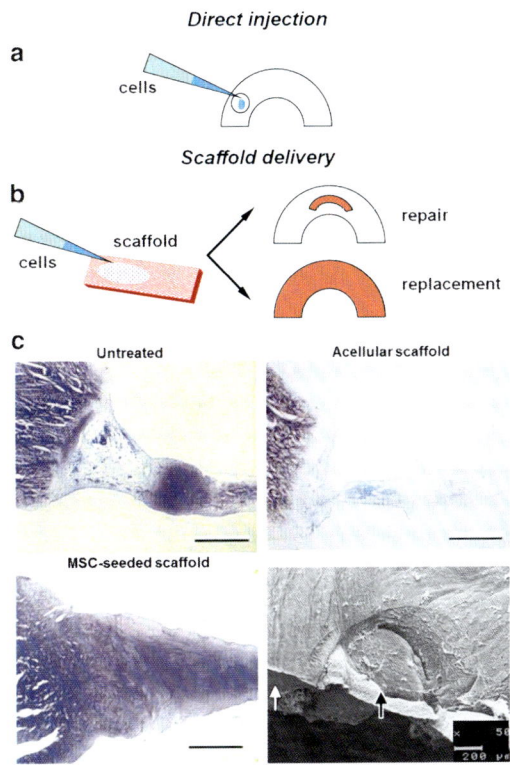

Fig. 10.4 Cellularity can be increased by (**a**) direct injection of cells into the lesion or (**b**) delivery via a scaffold. (**c**) Bone marrow-derived mesenchymal stem cells seeded onto a hyaluronan-collagen composite scaffold improved matrix production and integration in rabbits compared to untreated and acellular groups (reprinted with permission from John Wiley and Sons from reference [95]). SEM image shows the integrated interface of the tissue (*white arrow*) and pre-cultured scaffold (*black arrow*)

soluble factors and/or mechanical stimulation that promote anabolic activity and inhibit inflammation (Fig. 10.5). These experimental strategies to enhance integrative repair will be discussed in the following sections.

Methods to Enhance Vascularity in Meniscus Repair

Inability of the avascular, inner portion of the meniscus to heal has provided the impetus to investigate means to enhance vascularity via surgical approaches (Fig. 10.3). These approaches include mechanical rasping, trephination, and the introduction of vascularized grafts to the wound site. Partial removal of the wound interface by abrasion has been shown to encourage vascularization by inducing production and release of growth factors and cytokines beneficial to healing [36, 37]. This technique has been used experimentally to repair longitudinal meniscal tears of the avascular zone in rabbits and humans, although it was reported that success was dependent on the distance of the joint capsule to the tear site as well as the size and stability of the tear, indicating that proximity of a vascularized source was still necessary [38]. This problem can be addressed by creating vascular "access" channels that connect the inner zone to the peripheral vasculature (Fig. 10.3b). The provision of such a vascular conduit was pioneered separately by Gershuni et al. [39] and Zhang et al. [40, 41] in animal models. However, trephined channels are prone to collapse during normal physiologic loading, and the removal of meniscal cores can disrupt the aligned collagen fibers and further destabilize meniscal architecture. In a prospective study, Zhang et al. found that symptomatic re-tear rates decreased after combining arthroscopic trephination with suturing to ensure stability, but healing was not evaluated [42]. To maintain biomechanical integrity after core removal, Cook et al. developed a bioabsorbable conduit composed of poly(L-lactic) acid that allowed for fibrovascular tissue ingrowth, which proved superior to trephination alone in a canine model [43] (Fig. 10.3c). Alternatively, paramensical synovial abrasion can be applied to increase vascularity and provide chemotactic factors up to 5 mm from the outer meniscal rim [44]. Vascularized synovial flaps can also be placed within the meniscal defect to provide both a blood supply and a source of synoviocytes that can infiltrate the wound site and lay down matrix to bridge the gap [19, 39, 45, 46] (Fig. 10.3d). Indeed, interpositional free synovial autografts can improve integration in vitro despite these grafts lacking connections to the systemic vasculature in this model. This indicates that the mechanism of action may be in provision of an added source of regenerative cells or by the graft itself acting as a scaffold for cell migration [45, 47]. In fact, it

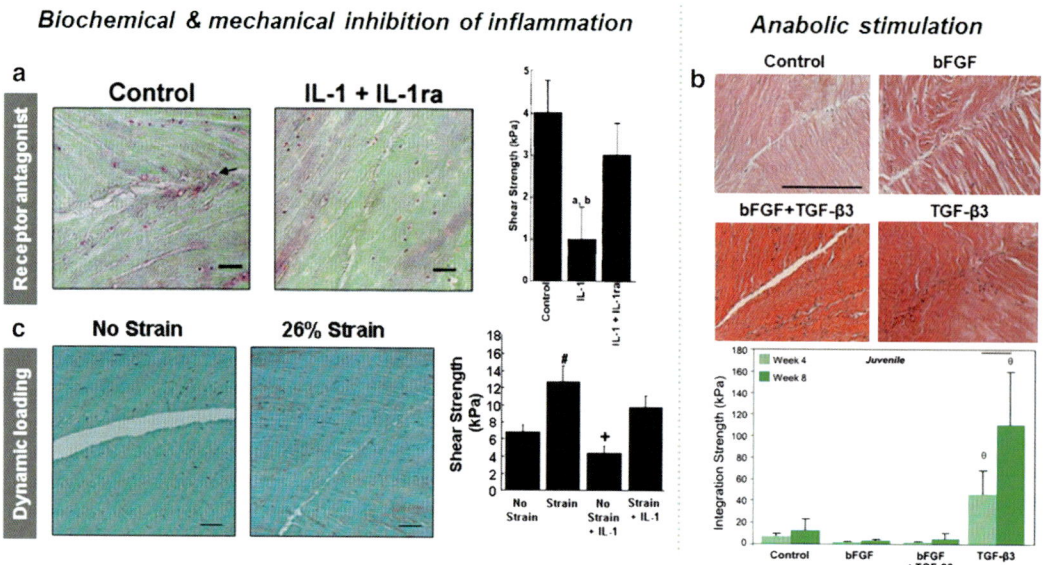

Fig. 10.5 Modification of the environment via biochemical and mechanical cues can augment integration. (**a**) The addition of IL-1 receptor antagonist (IL-1ra) in the presence of inflammatory cytokine IL-1 increases integrative shear strength of porcine meniscus in vitro (reprinted with permission from John Wiley and Sons from reference [32]). (**b**) Supplementation with the pro-matrix growth factor TGF-β3 improves integration strength of juvenile bovine meniscus in vitro, while addition of promitotic bFGF does not enhance repair, even when applied in conjunction with TGF-β3 [98]. (**c**) The application of dynamic loading increases integrative shear strength of porcine meniscus in vitro, overriding the catabolic effects of IL-1 (reprinted with permission from Elsevier from reference [34])

is thought that superficial cells of the meniscus originated from the synovium and that these cells may be implicated in meniscal healing [48, 49].

To enhance vascularity without surgically removing or introducing tissue, angiogenic factors such as vascular endothelial growth factor (VEGF) [50, 51] and angiogenin [52] have been utilized to promote neovascularization (new vessel formation) at the site of repair. VEGF is a potent endothelial cell chemokine and mitogen that induces formation of new capillaries when delivered at high concentrations [53], whereas angiogenin interacts with both endothelial and smooth muscle cells to promote formation of vascular structures [54]. Although angiogenin was found to promote neovascularization of the avascular zone in rabbits, two sheep studies investigating the application of VEGF released through poly(D,L-lactide) acid suture coatings concluded that local treatment with VEGF did not enhance meniscal angiogenesis or healing in either the vascular or avascular zone [50, 51] (Fig. 10.3e).

In these latter studies, the authors speculated that a longer duration of growth factor delivery, using a combination of several angiogenic factors involved in vessel wall assembly, may be necessary. These issues could be addressed by using a composite scaffold, where discrete components can be incorporated to release multiple bioactive factors with differing temporal release profiles [55]. For instance, Ionescu et al. recently developed an electrospun scaffold for fibrous connective tissue engineering that releases VEGF rapidly from water-soluble poly(ethylene oxide) nanofibers and gradually from embedded poly(lactic-co-glycolic acid) microspheres [56]. Using this versatile platform of gradual elution, a combination of VEGF, angiogenin, platelet-derived growth factor, and/or angiopoietin may be used to promote neovascularization.

Endogenous cells can also be acquired from the vasculature to increase cellularity and stimulate healing at the wound site, either via the introduction of a fibrin clot or through microfracture of the underlying bone. It has been argued that it is the hematoma and subsequent clotting, rather than the continuous bloody supply, that are critical to the induction of a repair response [57]. Acting as a source of reparative cells, growth factors, and temporary matrix, exogenous fibrin clots can be precipitated and inserted into meniscal defects to stimulate a healing response [58–62]. In a canine model, Arnockzy et al. found that meniscal defects filled with fibrin clots remodeled into fibrocartilage with chondroid cells after 6 months, although the reparative tissue could still be histologically distinguished from native tissue [58]. Clinical repair of acute, isolated meniscal tears, including complete radial tears that cross avascular regions, were also improved after clot injection [60, 62, 63]. Despite some experimental success, fibrin clots have not been widely adopted because they are difficult to place arthroscopically and are often destroyed or lost during the insertion process. To prevent loss after placement, the fibrin clot can be covered by a fascia sheath [61] or secured by a suture [64] (Fig. 10.3f). A minimally invasive intra-articular method to create a fibrin clot in situ was also developed to bypass the difficulty of clot acquisition and placement [65]. Similarly, an artificial hematoma can be created by releasing marrow elements into the joint space via microfracture of the intercondylar notch [66, 67] to expedite early recovery. To attract and protect endogenous fibrin clots and other host elements after hemarthrosis, small intestine submucosa grafts may be used to promote cellular attachment and expedite regeneration [68–71].

Methods to Improve Cellularity in Meniscus Repair

While strategies for enhancing vascularization are promising, a more established approach is to harvest and deliver therapeutic cells to the wound site, independent of the blood supply (Fig. 10.4). Cells can be recruited from adjacent tissues, injected directly into the lesion, or delivered via a scaffold to improve the intrinsically low cellularity of the native tissue. Ideally, cells should be autologous and abundant, easily acquired and

expanded in vitro, and able to produce fibrocartilaginous matrix [72]. The success of autologous chondrocyte implantation (ACI) for cartilage repair demonstrates that cell therapy is clinically feasible and could be adapted to improve meniscus repair. Of particular interest for such applications are synoviocytes, chondrocytes, and meniscal cells, as well as multipotent mesenchymal stem cells (MSCs) that can differentiate into a meniscal-like cell phenotype.

Located just adjacent to the meniscus, fibroblast-like type B synoviocytes produce matrix proteins such as collagen and hyaluronan for the intimal interstitium [73]. Studies by Arnoczky et al. [74] have demonstrated that these cells can cross the synovio-meniscal boundary to reach the wound site and contribute to the repair process. It is also likely that cells of synovial origin play a role in integrating free synovial grafts [45, 47] as well as repopulating meniscal allografts [75, 76]. To that end, parameniscal abrasion of the synovial intima may liberate these cells and expedite their migration to the defect [77]. On the other hand, chondrocytes are typically harvested from articular cartilage, expanded in vitro, and delivered to the lesion site seeded inside a biocompatible scaffold. When inserted into a defect, allogenic chondrocytes improved bonding of the meniscal margins by depositing cartilaginous matrix that integrated the scaffold, in this case devitalized meniscus, with the native tissue [78]. In a more recent integration study, Weinand et al. found that auricular chondrocytes seeded onto Vicryl meshes may provide more healing capacity than articular chondrocytes due to increased production of elastin [79]. Unlike synoviocytes and chondrocytes, meniscal cells have been evaluated more for their use in engineering replacement tissue than for their role in directly modulating repair. Nevertheless, due to their ability to deposit fibrocartilage when seeded onto 3D scaffolds, meniscal cells have potential to be used in the same way as chondrocytes for integrative repair [80–84]. Interestingly, the ability of meniscal cells to produce ECM in vitro does not decrease with age, making meniscal surgical debris a potential source of viable cells for implantation [83].

Another source of regenerative cells for meniscus repair applications is undifferentiated mesenchymal stem cell (MSCs). These cells are capable of differentiating into chondrocytes or cells of other mesodermal lineage if provided the appropriate biochemical and mechanical cues. MSCs can be obtained from several sources, including bone marrow, synovium, and adipose tissue, thus bypassing the need to harvest meniscal or chondral tissue to isolate autologous cells. The most common technique for MSC delivery is injection either into the joint space or directly into the tear site, which is then often closed with sutures (Fig. 10.4a). Abdel-Hamid et al. found that injection of bone marrow MSCs into a meniscal tear in a canine model improved healing by promoting angiogenesis, chondrogenesis, and collagen fiber deposition [85]. In rat and rabbit models, fluorescently labeled synovial-derived MSCs injected into the joint space filled meniscal defects and differentiated into chondrocytes that produced type II collagen [86–88]. Adipose-derived MSCs produced similar regenerative effects when injected directly into avascular meniscal lesions in rabbits [89]. The first human case of autologous MSC transplantation for meniscal cartilage regeneration was done via percutaneous intra-articular injection [90]. Bone marrow-derived MSCs were harvested from the iliac crest, expanded in vitro, and injected into the joint space of an osteoarthritic knee. Analysis via MRI showed evidence of increased meniscal volume after 3 months, although a biopsy was not performed to determine the composition of the new tissue.

Despite the promise of cell therapy, it is often difficult to localize or retain cells at the lesion using injection alone. A study by Agung et al. tracking intra-articular injected bone marrow MSCs with green fluorescent protein (GFP) found that MSCs must be delivered in high numbers (1×10^7) for them to actively mobilize to the meniscus and generate extracellular matrix at the site of injury. However, this high concentration of cells also caused the formation of unwanted scar tissue [91] and may result in the undesirable colonization of surrounding structures. Consequently, it may be more effective to localize cell delivery to the region of interest with the use of a pre-seeded biodegradable scaffold (Fig. 10.4b). For example, fluorescent tracking of transplanted MSCs that were embedded in fibrin glue demonstrated retention of cells inside the meniscal defect [92, 93]. Other successful biomaterials that have been used include collagen scaffolds [94] and hyaluronan-collagen composites [95] (Fig. 10.4c). It is important to note that while pre-culture of cells may generate fibrocartilage and thus improve mechanical properties, formation of new tissue also could inhibit integration of the scaffold in vivo [95, 96]. Thus, while there are still many factors to optimize for cell-based treatments, there is strong evidence that viable autologous cells, and MSCs in particular, can significantly augment meniscal healing.

Influence of Soluble Factors on Meniscus Repair

The presence of viable cells at the wound site does not in and of itself guarantee a robust repair response. To expedite the healing process, cells should be in a noninflammatory, instructive environment that encourages proliferation and synthesis of extracellular matrix. McNulty et al. demonstrated that inhibition of inflammatory cytokines IL-1β and TNFα with IL-1 receptor antagonist (IL-1ra) and anti-TNFα monoclonal antibody (TNFα mAB), respectively, as well as inhibition of broad-spectrum matrix metalloproteinase (MMP) activity, improved the integration strength of meniscal explants in vitro [32, 33] (Fig. 10.5a and Table 10.1). MMP inhibitors, such as tetracycline, hold promise as agents which may potentiate meniscal healing. Conversely, growth factors such as transforming growth factor beta (TGF-β) [97–102], platelet-derived growth factor AB (PDGF-AB) [99, 102–106], insulin-like growth factor 1 (IGF-1) [99, 100, 102, 106, 107], and basic fibroblast growth factor (bFGF) [57, 99, 100, 108, 109] have been investigated for their mitogenic and anabolic effects on meniscal cells (Table 10.1). Since integrative strength is correlated with collagen deposition and cross-linking [110], the most significant improvement occurs

Table 10.1 Biologic factors of interest for meniscal repair and their effect on meniscal cell behavior and impact on integrative potential

Growth factor	Cellular effect	Integrative potential	Methods
TGF-β	Potent stimulator of matrix deposition	Increased	Monolayer [97, 100, 102], explant [97–99, 101], scaffold [98]
PDGF-AB	Intermediate stimulator of matrix deposition, proliferation, and migration	No data	Monolayer [102, 104, 106], explant [99, 103, 105]
IGF-1			Monolayer [100, 102, 106, 107], explant [99]
bFGF	Potent stimulator of proliferation	No effect	Monolayer [57, 100, 102, 108], explant [98, 99, 109], scaffold [98]
Inflammatory inhibitor	Cellular/environmental effect	Integrative potential	Method
IL-1ra	Receptor antagonist competitively blocks IL-1 receptor	Increased	Explant [32]
Anti-TNF mAB	Monoclonal antibody binds and inhibits TNFα	Increased	Explant [32]
MMP inhibitor GM 6001	Broad-spectrum MMP inhibitor	Increased	Explant [33]

when ECM synthesis increases as a result of growth factor stimulation. Throughout the literature, the most successful growth factor for increasing cell division and proteoglycan and collagen production in cell cultures and tissue explants in vitro is TGF-β1 [99]. McNulty et al. found that TGF-β1 supplementation increases the interfacial shear strength of meniscal explants enough to overcome the catabolic effects of IL-1-mediated MMP activity [101]. TGF-β3 has also been investigated for its pro-matrix effects and has been shown to improve the integration of juvenile and adult meniscal explants when delivered continuously over time in vitro [98] (Fig. 10.5b). Growth factors of intermediate efficacy include PDGF-AB and IGF-1 [99]. PDGF-AB also induces meniscal cell migration [106] as well as proteoglycan production [99, 105], making it an attractive agent for recruiting endogenous cells to the wound margin. However, a region-specific response to PDGF-AB has been reported, where proliferation increased within meniscal explants from the peripheral zone but not so in the central region, possibly due to local variation in growth factor receptors [103]. Subsequent studies found that meniscal cells from all zones show a proliferative response in monolayer culture, suggesting that regional matrix sequestration of soluble factors may be the cause instead [104, 106]. IGF-1 supplementation similarly enhances cellularity and ECM synthesis and is especially stimulatory for cells in the inner avascular zone [107]. Less successful have been growth factors that stimulate proliferation but little to no increase in matrix protein production, such as bFGF [57, 98–100, 102, 108], perhaps because less resources are devoted to repair when cells are in a mitotic state (Fig. 10.5b). In this case, it may be beneficial to deliver a mitogen over the short term, coupled with sustained delivery of a pro-matrix growth factor either via drug-releasing scaffolds or sutures, or gene transfer to ensure long-term stability.

Influence of Mechanical Factors on Meniscus Repair

Inflammation and matrix production, and therefore the repair outcome, is also mechano-responsive. Meniscal cell gene expression controlling the balance of structural protein synthesis and degradation can be altered by mechanical stimuli, such as tensile and compressive loading. Meniscal cells in monolayer respond to cyclic biaxial stretch by increasing matrix protein biosynthesis [111]. MSCs cultured in nanofibrous scaffolds respond similarly to dynamic tensile loading, with improvements in matrix production and tensile modulus in engineered fibrocartilage [112]. In studies done with meniscal explants, static but not dynamic compression increased MMP activity and inhibited matrix production, even in the presence of anabolic growth factors [35, 99]. In fact, cyclic loading was required for meniscal homeostasis [113] and treatment with dynamic compression antagonized the catabolic effects of IL-1-mediated MMP degradation and consequent glycosaminoglycan release in meniscal explants [34] (Fig. 10.5c). Nonetheless, overloading the meniscus at high strains (10–20 %) [114] or high strain rates (50 %/s) may cause cell lysis and tissue damage that is physically undetectable [115]. These studies clearly show that the mechanical environment can synergize with the biochemical environment to promote (or delay) repair, depending on the duration and degree of loading applied.

These effects of mechanical forces on meniscal repair are also seen in vivo. For instance, prolonged cast immobilization prevented collagen production in a canine model, indicating that normal joint mobility is essential for meniscal healing [116]. Furthermore, immobilization significantly reduced blood flow post-injury in rabbits and promoted menisci degeneration [117–119]. A sheep study yielded similar findings, where weight-bearing menisci supported more load than those that were immobilized after suture repair [120]. Collectively, these results suggest that controlled mobilization should be initiated as soon as possible after repair to encourage long-term healing of isolated lesions, although rehabilitation should be passive or at a low, controlled intensity to prevent tear destabilization and intra-articular damage in the immediate postoperative period.

Summary and Conclusions

As the negative sequelae of meniscectomy become clearer, development of novel methods aimed at the biologic augmentation of meniscal healing has increased tremendously in recent years. Other emerging approaches that aim to enhance repair include high-frequency stimulation [121], partial enzymatic degradation of the wound margin [122], and pro-matrix gene therapy [102, 123]. The advancement of biocompatible scaffolds, either as a vehicle for delivering cells and/or bioactive molecules or as engineered meniscal replacements, is also highly promising. Such tissue-engineered constructs could be used to replace large portions of resected degenerate tissue injured beyond physical repair. Already, two synthetic implants have been clinically approved for use in Europe, one composed of collagen (collagen meniscus implant (CMI), Ivy Sports Medicine LLC) and the other polyurethane (Actifit®, Orteq Ltd) [124]. However, these implants are not tailored to match individual patient dimensions nor do their microstructures replicate the mechanical anisotropy seen in native meniscus. Novel approaches to generate anatomically correct structures have recently emerged, including the use of image-guided injection molding to replicate meniscus geometry [125] and the electrospinning of circumferentially oriented nanofibers to mimic collagen alignment and mechanical properties [126]. These engineered constructs offer promise for replacement when endogenous repair cannot resolve the meniscal injury.

Regardless of the specific technique or application (improvement of repair or replacement of damaged tissue), future directions will increasingly focus on combining minimally invasive surgical stabilization with cell therapy and stimulatory environmental cues to encourage vascularization and integration at the lesion site. As these experimental methods for avascular tear repair become clinically available, the current standard of partial meniscal removal will be shifted towards a paradigm of preservation and regeneration. This transition towards regeneration and/or functional replacement rather than simple removal has the potential to dramatically improve long-term joint health in the many thousands of patients who suffer from the sequelae of acute and degenerative meniscus pathology.

Acknowledgments This work was supported by the National Institutes of Health (R01 AR056624), the Department of Veterans Affairs (I01 RX000174), the Penn

Center for Musculoskeletal Disorders, and the Musculoskeletal Transplant Foundation. The views expressed in this article are those of the authors and do not necessarily reflect the position or policy of the National Institutes of Health, Department of Veterans Affairs, or the US government.

References

1. Shrive NG, O'Connor JJ, Goodfellow JW. Load-bearing in the knee joint. Clin Orthop Relat Res. 1978;131:279–87.
2. Fithian DC, Kelly MA, Mow VC. Material properties and structure–function relationships in the menisci. Clin Orthop Relat Res. 1990;252:19–31.
3. Hede A, Larsen E, Sandberg H. The long term outcome of open total and partial meniscectomy related to the quantity and site of the meniscus removed. Int Orthop. 1992;16(2):122–5.
4. Nielsen AB, Yde J. Epidemiology of acute knee injuries: a prospective hospital investigation. J Trauma. 1991;31(12):1644–8.
5. Arendt EA. Orthopaedic knowledge update: sports medicine 2. Rosemont, IL: American Academy of Orthopaedic Surgeons; 1999.
6. Boyd KT, Myers PT. Meniscus preservation; rationale, repair techniques and results. Knee. 2003;10(1):1–11.
7. DeHaven KE. Meniscus repair. Am J Sports Med. 1999;27(2):242–50.
8. Morgan CD, Wojtys EM, Casscells CD, Casscells SW. Arthroscopic meniscal repair evaluated by second-look arthroscopy. Am J Sports Med. 1991;19(6):632–7. discussion 7–8.
9. Eggli S, Wegmuller H, Kosina J, Huckell C, Jakob RP. Long-term results of arthroscopic meniscal repair. An analysis of isolated tears. Am J Sports Med. 1995;23(6):715–20.
10. Miller Jr DB. Arthroscopic meniscus repair. Am J Sports Med. 1988;16(4):315–20.
11. Hanks GA, Gause TM, Sebastianelli WJ, O'Donnell CS, Kalenak A. Repair of peripheral meniscal tears: open versus arthroscopic technique. Arthroscopy. 1991;7(1):72–7.
12. Rubman MH, Noyes FR, Barber-Westin SD. Arthroscopic repair of meniscal tears that extend into the avascular zone. A review of 198 single and complex tears. Am J Sports Med. 1998;26(1):87–95.
13. Aagaard H, Verdonk R. Function of the normal meniscus and consequences of meniscal resection. Scand J Med Sci Sports. 1999;9(3):134–40.
14. Englund M. Meniscal tear: a feature of osteoarthritis. Acta Orthop Scand Suppl. 2004;75(312):1–45.
15. Day B, Mackenzie WG, Shim SS, Leung G. The vascular and nerve supply of the human meniscus. Arthroscopy. 1985;1(1):58–62.
16. Arnoczky SP, Warren RF. Microvasculature of the human meniscus. Am J Sports Med. 1982;10(2):90–5.
17. King D. The function of semilunar cartilages. J Bone Joint Surg Am. 1936;18(4):1069–76.
18. Arnoczky SP, Warren RF. The microvasculature of the meniscus and its response to injury. An experimental study in the dog. Am J Sports Med. 1983;11(3):131–41.
19. Ghadially FN, Wedge JH, Lalonde JM. Experimental methods of repairing injured menisci. J Bone Joint Surg Br. 1986;68(1):106–10.
20. Heatley FW. The meniscus—can it be repaired? An experimental investigation in rabbits. J Bone Joint Surg Br. 1980;62(3):397–402.
21. Noyes FR, Barber-Westin SD. Management of meniscus tears that extend into the avascular region. Clin Sports Med. 2012;31(1):65–90.
22. Greis PE, Bardana DD, Holmstrom MC, Burks RT. Meniscal injury: I. Basic science and evaluation. J Am Acad Orthop Surg. 2002;10(3):168–76.
23. Clark CR, Ogden JA. Development of the menisci of the human knee joint. Morphological changes and their potential role in childhood meniscal injury. J Bone Joint Surg Am. 1983;65(4):538–47.
24. Ionescu LC, Lee GC, Garcia GH, Zachry TL, Shah RP, Sennett BJ, et al. Maturation state-dependent alterations in meniscus integration: implications for scaffold design and tissue engineering. Tissue Eng Part A. 2011;17(1–2):193–204.
25. Mesiha M, Zurakowski D, Soriano J, Nielson JH, Zarins B, Murray MM. Pathologic characteristics of the torn human meniscus. Am J Sports Med. 2007;35(1):103–12.
26. Kobayashi K, Fujimoto E, Deie M, Sumen Y, Ikuta Y, Ochi M. Regional differences in the healing potential of the meniscus—an organ culture model to eliminate the influence of microvasculature and the synovium. Knee. 2004;11(4):271–8.
27. Upton ML, Chen J, Setton LA. Region-specific constitutive gene expression in the adult porcine meniscus. J Orthop Res. 2006;24(7):1562–70.
28. McDevitt CA, Murkherjee S, Kambic H, Parker R. Emerging concepts of the cell biology of the meniscus. Curr Opin Orthop. 2002;13:345–50.
29. Hellio Le Graverand MP, Ou Y, Schield-Yee T, Barclay L, Hart D, Natsume T, et al. The cells of the rabbit meniscus: their arrangement, interrelationship, morphological variations and cytoarchitecture. J Anat. 2001;198(5):525–35.
30. Fuller ES, Smith MM, Little CB, Melrose J. Zonal differences in meniscus matrix turnover and cytokine response. Osteoarthritis Cartilage. 2012;20(1):49–59.
31. McDevitt CA, Webber RJ. The ultrastructure and biochemistry of meniscal cartilage. Clin Orthop Relat Res. 1992;252:8–18.
32. McNulty AL, Moutos FT, Weinberg JB, Guilak F. Enhanced integrative repair of the porcine meniscus in vitro by inhibition of interleukin-1 or tumor necrosis factor alpha. Arthritis Rheum. 2007;56(9):3033–42.
33. McNulty AL, Weinberg JB, Guilak F. Inhibition of matrix metalloproteinases enhances in vitro repair of

the meniscus. Clin Orthop Relat Res. 2009; 467(6):1557–67.

34. McNulty AL, Estes BT, Wilusz RE, Weinberg JB, Guilak F. Dynamic loading enhances integrative meniscal repair in the presence of interleukin-1. Osteoarthritis Cartilage. 2010;18(6):830–8.

35. Upton ML, Chen J, Guilak F, Setton LA. Differential effects of static and dynamic compression on meniscal cell gene expression. J Orthop Res. 2003;21(6): 963–9.

36. Okuda K, Ochi M, Shu N, Uchio Y. Meniscal rasping for repair of meniscal tear in the avascular zone. Arthroscopy. 1999;15(3):281–6.

37. Ochi M, Uchio Y, Okuda K, Shu N, Yamaguchi H, Sakai Y. Expression of cytokines after meniscal rasping to promote meniscal healing. Arthroscopy. 2001;17(7):724–31.

38. Uchio Y, Ochi M, Adachi N, Kawasaki K, Iwasa J. Results of rasping of meniscal tears with and without anterior cruciate ligament injury as evaluated by second-look arthroscopy. Arthroscopy. 2003;19(5): 463–9.

39. Gershuni DH, Skyhar MJ, Danzig LA, Camp J, Hargens AR, Akeson WH. Experimental models to promote healing of tears in the avascular segment of canine knee menisci. J Bone Joint Surg Am. 1989;71(9):1363–70.

40. Zhang ZN, Tu KY, Xu YK, Zhang WM, Liu ZT, Ou SH. Treatment of longitudinal injuries in avascular area of meniscus in dogs by trephination. Arthroscopy. 1988;4(3):151–9.

41. Zhang Z, Arnold JA, Williams T, McCann B. Repairs by trephination and suturing of longitudinal injuries in the avascular area of the meniscus in goats. Am J Sports Med. 1995;23(1):35–41.

42. Zhang Z, Arnold JA. Trephination and suturing of avascular meniscal tears: a clinical study of the trephination procedure. Arthroscopy. 1996;12(6):726–31.

43. Cook JL, Fox DB. A novel bioabsorbable conduit augments healing of avascular meniscal tears in a dog model. Am J Sports Med. 2007;35(11):1877–87.

44. Henning CE, Lynch MA, Clark JR. Vascularity for healing of meniscus repairs. Arthroscopy. 1987; 3(1):13–8.

45. Ochi M, Mochizuki Y, Deie M, Ikuta Y. Augmented meniscal healing with free synovial autografts: an organ culture model. Arch Orthop Trauma Surg. 1996;115(3–4):123–6.

46. Jitsuiki J, Ochi M, Ikuta Y. Meniscal repair enhanced by an interpositional free synovial autograft: an experimental study in rabbits. Arthroscopy. 1994; 10(6):659–66.

47. Yamazaki K, Tachibana Y. Vascularized synovial flap promoting regeneration of the cryopreserved meniscal allograft: experimental study in rabbits. J Orthop Sci. 2003;8(1):62–8.

48. Kambic HE, Futani H, McDevitt CA. Cell, matrix changes and alpha-smooth muscle actin expression in repair of the canine meniscus. Wound Repair Regen. 2000;8(6):554–61.

49. Hu SY, Wang S, Zuo RT, Wang KL, Qin L. Meniscus and synovial membrane: an electron microscopic study on rabbits. Can J Appl Physiol. 2001;26(3):254–60.

50. Petersen W, Pufe T, Starke C, Fuchs T, Kopf S, Neumann W, et al. The effect of locally applied vascular endothelial growth factor on meniscus healing: gross and histological findings. Arch Orthop Trauma Surg. 2007;127(4):235–40.

51. Kopf S, Birkenfeld F, Becker R, Petersen W, Starke C, Wruck CJ, et al. Local treatment of meniscal lesions with vascular endothelial growth factor. J Bone Joint Surg Am. 2010;92(16):2682–91.

52. King TV, Vallee BL. Neovascularisation of the meniscus with angiogenin. An experimental study in rabbits. J Bone Joint Surg Br. 1991;73(4):587–90.

53. Phillips GD, Stone AM, Jones BD, Schultz JC, Whitehead RA, Knighton DR. Vascular endothelial growth factor (rhVEGF165) stimulates direct angiogenesis in the rabbit cornea. In Vivo. 1994;8(6):961–5.

54. Gao X, Xu Z. Mechanisms of action of angiogenin. Acta Biochim Biophys Sin (Shanghai). 2008;40(7): 619–24.

55. Richardson TP, Peters MC, Ennett AB, Mooney DJ. Polymeric system for dual growth factor delivery. Nat Biotechnol. 2001;19(11):1029–34.

56. Ionescu LC, Fisher MB, Schenker ML, Esterhai JL, Mauck RL. VEGF delivery from electrospun composites increases vascular density in vivo. Orthopaedic Research Society annual meeting 2012. Abstract #0634.

57. Webber RJ, Harris MG, Hough Jr AJ. Cell culture of rabbit meniscal fibrochondrocytes: proliferative and synthetic response to growth factors and ascorbate. J Orthop Res. 1985;3(1):36–42.

58. Arnoczky SP, Warren RF, Spivak JM. Meniscal repair using an exogenous fibrin clot. An experimental study in dogs. J Bone Joint Surg Am. 1988;70(8):1209–17.

59. Nakhostine M, Gershuni DH, Danzig LA. Effects of an in-substance conduit with injection of a blood clot on tears in the avascular region of the meniscus. Acta Orthop Belg. 1991;57(3):242–6.

60. Henning CE, Lynch MA, Yearout KM, Vequist SW, Stallbaumer RJ, Decker KA. Arthroscopic meniscal repair using an exogenous fibrin clot. Clin Orthop Relat Res. 1990;252:64–72.

61. Henning CE, Yearout KM, Vequist SW, Stallbaumer RJ, Decker KA. Use of the fascia sheath coverage and exogenous fibrin clot in the treatment of complex meniscal tears. Am J Sports Med. 1991;19(6):626–31.

62. van Trommel MF, Simonian PT, Potter HG, Wickiewicz TL. Arthroscopic meniscal repair with fibrin clot of complete radial tears of the lateral meniscus in the avascular zone. Arthroscopy. 1998; 14(4):360–5.

63. Ra HJ, Ha JK, Jang SH, Lee DW, Kim JG. Arthroscopic inside-out repair of complete radial tears of the meniscus with a fibrin clot. Knee Surg Sports Traumatol Arthrosc. 2012. doi:10.1007/s00167-012-2191-3. Print ISSN: 0942–2056. Online ISSN: 1433–7347.

64. Jang SH, Ha JK, Lee DW, Kim JG. Fibrin clot delivery system for meniscal repair. Knee Surg Relat Res. 2011;23(3):180–3.

65. Sethi PM, Cooper A, Jokl P. Technical tips in orthopaedics: meniscal repair with use of an in situ fibrin clot. Arthroscopy. 2003;19(5):E44.

66. Freedman KB, Nho SJ, Cole BJ. Marrow stimulating technique to augment meniscus repair. Arthroscopy. 2003;19(7):794–8.

67. Driscoll MD, Robin BN, Horie M, Hubert ZT, Sampson HW, Jupiter DC, et al. Marrow stimulation improves meniscal healing at early endpoints in a rabbit meniscal injury model. Arthroscopy. 2013; 29(1):113–21.

68. Cook JL, Fox DB, Malaviya P, Tomlinson JL, Kuroki K, Cook CR, et al. Long-term outcome for large meniscal defects treated with small intestinal submucosa in a dog model. Am J Sports Med. 2006; 34(1):32–42.

69. Fox DB, Cook JL, Arnoczky SP, Tomlinson JL, Kuroki K, Kreeger JM, et al. Fibrochondrogenesis of free intraarticular small intestinal submucosa scaffolds. Tissue Eng. 2004;10(1–2):129–37.

70. Bradley MP, Fadale PD, Hulstyn MJ, Muirhead WR, Lifrak JT. Porcine small intestine submucosa for repair of goat meniscal defects. Orthopedics. 2007; 30(8):650–6.

71. Gastel JA, Muirhead WR, Lifrak JT, Fadale PD, Hulstyn MJ, Labrador DP. Meniscal tissue regeneration using a collagenous biomaterial derived from porcine small intestine submucosa. Arthroscopy. 2001;17(2):151–9.

72. Hoben GM, Athanasiou KA. Meniscal repair with fibrocartilage engineering. Sports Med Arthrosc. 2006;14(3):129–37.

73. Iwanaga T, Shikichi M, Kitamura H, Yanase H, Nozawa-Inoue K. Morphology and functional roles of synoviocytes in the joint. Arch Histol Cytol. 2000;63(1):17–31.

74. Arnoczky SP, Warren RF, Kaplan N. Meniscal remodeling following partial meniscectomy—an experimental study in the dog. Arthroscopy. 1985;1(4):247–52.

75. Arnoczky SP, DiCarlo EF, O'Brien SJ, Warren RF. Cellular repopulation of deep-frozen meniscal autografts: an experimental study in the dog. Arthroscopy. 1992;8(4):428–36.

76. Rodeo SA, Seneviratne A, Suzuki K, Felker K, Wickiewicz TL, Warren RF. Histological analysis of human meniscal allografts. A preliminary report. J Bone Joint Surg Am. 2000;82-A(8):1071–82.

77. Nakhostine M, Gershuni DH, Anderson R, Danzig LA, Weiner GM. Effects of abrasion therapy on tears in the avascular region of sheep menisci. Arthroscopy. 1990;6(4):280–7.

78. Peretti GM, Gill TJ, Xu JW, Randolph MA, Morse KR, Zaleske DJ. Cell-based therapy for meniscal repair: a large animal study. Am J Sports Med. 2004;32(1):146–58.

79. Weinand C, Peretti GM, Adams Jr SB, Randolph MA, Savvidis E, Gill TJ. Healing potential of transplanted allogeneic chondrocytes of three different sources in lesions of the avascular zone of the meniscus: a pilot study. Arch Orthop Trauma Surg. 2006;126(9):599–605.

80. Nakata K, Shino K, Hamada M, Mae T, Miyama T, Shinjo H, et al. Human meniscus cell: characterization of the primary culture and use for tissue engineering. Clin Orthop Relat Res. 2001;391 Suppl: S208–18.

81. Mueller SM, Shortkroff S, Schneider TO, Breinan HA, Yannas IV, Spector M. Meniscus cells seeded in type I and type II collagen-GAG matrices in vitro. Biomaterials. 1999;20(8):701–9.

82. Ibarra C, Koski JA, Warren RF. Tissue engineering meniscus: cells and matrix. Orthop Clin North Am. 2000;31(3):411–8.

83. Baker BM, Nathan AS, Huffman GR, Mauck RL. Tissue engineering with meniscus cells derived from surgical debris. Osteoarthritis Cartilage. 2009;17(3):336–45.

84. Freymann U, Endres M, Neumann K, Scholman HJ, Morawietz L, Kaps C. Expanded human meniscus-derived cells in 3-D polymer-hyaluronan scaffolds for meniscus repair. Acta Biomater. 2012;8(2): 677–85.

85. Abdel-Hamid M, Hussein MR, Ahmad AF, Elgezawi EM. Enhancement of the repair of meniscal wounds in the red–white zone (middle third) by the injection of bone marrow cells in canine animal model. Int J Exp Pathol. 2005;86(2):117–23.

86. Mizuno K, Muneta T, Morito T, Ichinose S, Koga H, Nimura A, et al. Exogenous synovial stem cells adhere to defect of meniscus and differentiate into cartilage cells. J Med Dent Sci. 2008;55(1):101–11.

87. Horie M, Sekiya I, Muneta T, Ichinose S, Matsumoto K, Saito H, et al. Intra-articular Injected synovial stem cells differentiate into meniscal cells directly and promote meniscal regeneration without mobilization to distant organs in rat massive meniscal defect. Stem Cells. 2009;27(4):878–87.

88. Horie M, Driscoll MD, Sampson HW, Sekiya I, Caroom CT, Prockop DJ, et al. Implantation of allogenic synovial stem cells promotes meniscal regeneration in a rabbit meniscal defect model. J Bone Joint Surg Am. 2012;94(8):701–12.

89. Ruiz-Iban MA, Diaz-Heredia J, Garcia-Gomez I, Gonzalez-Lizan F, Elias-Martin E, Abraira V. The effect of the addition of adipose-derived mesenchymal stem cells to a meniscal repair in the avascular zone: an experimental study in rabbits. Arthroscopy. 2011;27(12):1688–96.

90. Centeno CJ, Busse D, Kisiday J, Keohan C, Freeman M, Karli D. Regeneration of meniscus cartilage in a knee treated with percutaneously implanted autologous mesenchymal stem cells. Med Hypotheses. 2008;71(6):900–8.

91. Agung M, Ochi M, Yanada S, Adachi N, Izuta Y, Yamasaki T, et al. Mobilization of bone marrow-derived mesenchymal stem cells into the injured tissues after intraarticular injection and their

contribution to tissue regeneration. Knee Surg Sports Traumatol Arthrosc. 2006;14(12):1307–14.

92. Dutton AQ, Choong PF, Goh JC, Lee EH, Hui JH. Enhancement of meniscal repair in the avascular zone using mesenchymal stem cells in a porcine model. J Bone Joint Surg Br. 2010;92(1):169–75.

93. Izuta Y, Ochi M, Adachi N, Deie M, Yamasaki T, Shinomiya R. Meniscal repair using bone marrow-derived mesenchymal stem cells: experimental study using green fluorescent protein transgenic rats. Knee. 2005;12(3):217–23.

94. Pabbruwe MB, Kafienah W, Tarlton JF, Mistry S, Fox DJ, Hollander AP. Repair of meniscal cartilage white zone tears using a stem cell/collagen-scaffold implant. Biomaterials. 2010;31(9):2583–91.

95. Zellner J, Mueller M, Berner A, Dienstknecht T, Kujat R, Nerlich M, et al. Role of mesenchymal stem cells in tissue engineering of meniscus. J Biomed Mater Res A. 2010;94(4):1150–61.

96. Ionescu LC, Mauck RL. Porosity and cell preseeding influence electrospun scaffold maturation and meniscus integration in vitro. Tissue Eng Part A. 2013;19(3–4):538–47.

97. Collier S, Ghosh P. Effects of transforming growth factor beta on proteoglycan synthesis by cell and explant cultures derived from the knee joint meniscus. Osteoarthritis Cartilage. 1995;3(2):127–38.

98. Ionescu LC, Lee GC, Huang KL, Mauck RL. Growth factor supplementation improves native and engineered meniscus repair in vitro. Acta Biomater. 2012;8(10):3687–94.

99. Imler SM, Doshi AN, Levenston ME. Combined effects of growth factors and static mechanical compression on meniscus explant biosynthesis. Osteoarthritis Cartilage. 2004;12(9):736–44.

100. Esparza R, Gortazar AR, Forriol F. Cell study of the three areas of the meniscus: effect of growth factors in an experimental model in sheep. J Orthop Res. 2012;30(10):1647–51.

101. McNulty AL, Guilak F. Integrative repair of the meniscus: lessons from in vitro studies. Biorheology. 2008;45(3–4):487–500.

102. Kasemkijwattana C, Menetrey J, Goto H, Niyibizi C, Fu FH, Huard J. The use of growth factors, gene therapy and tissue engineering to improve meniscal healing. Mater Sci Eng C. 2000;13(1):19–28.

103. Spindler KP, Mayes CE, Miller RR, Imro AK, Davidson JM. Regional mitogenic response of the meniscus to platelet-derived growth factor (PDGF-AB). J Orthop Res. 1995;13(2):201–7.

104. Tumia NS, Johnstone AJ. Platelet derived growth factor-AB enhances knee meniscal cell activity in vitro. Knee. 2009;16(1):73–6.

105. Lietman SA, Hobbs W, Inoue N, Reddi AH. Effects of selected growth factors on porcine meniscus in chemically defined medium. Orthopedics. 2003;26(8):799–803.

106. Bhargava MM, Attia ET, Murrell GA, Dolan MM, Warren RF, Hannafin JA. The effect of cytokines on the proliferation and migration of bovine meniscal cells. Am J Sports Med. 1999;27(5):636–43.

107. Tumia NS, Johnstone AJ. Regional regenerative potential of meniscal cartilage exposed to recombinant insulin-like growth factor-I in vitro. J Bone Joint Surg Br. 2004;86(7):1077–81.

108. Tumia NS, Johnstone AJ. Promoting the proliferative and synthetic activity of knee meniscal fibrochondrocytes using basic fibroblast growth factor in vitro. Am J Sports Med. 2004;32(4):915–20.

109. Narita A, Takahara M, Ogino T, Fukushima S, Kimura Y, Tabata Y. Effect of gelatin hydrogel incorporating fibroblast growth factor 2 on human meniscal cells in an organ culture model. Knee. 2009;16(4):285–9.

110. DiMicco MA, Waters SN, Akeson WH, Sah RL. Integrative articular cartilage repair: dependence on developmental stage and collagen metabolism. Osteoarthritis Cartilage. 2002;10(3):218–25.

111. Upton ML, Hennerbichler A, Fermor B, Guilak F, Weinberg JB, Setton LA. Biaxial strain effects on cells from the inner and outer regions of the meniscus. Connect Tissue Res. 2006;47(4):207–14.

112. Baker BM, Shah RP, Huang AH, Mauck RL. Dynamic tensile loading improves the functional properties of mesenchymal stem cell-laden nanofiber-based fibrocartilage. Tissue Eng Part A. 2011;17(9–10):1445–55.

113. Natsu-Ume T, Majima T, Reno C, Shrive NG, Frank CB, Hart DA. Menisci of the rabbit knee require mechanical loading to maintain homeostasis: cyclic hydrostatic compression in vitro prevents derepression of catabolic genes. J Orthop Sci. 2005;10(4):396–405.

114. Zielinska B, Killian M, Kadmiel M, Nelsen M, Haut Donahue TL. Meniscal tissue explants response depends on level of dynamic compressive strain. Osteoarthritis Cartilage. 2009;17(6):754–60.

115. Nishimuta JF, Levenston ME. Response of cartilage and meniscus tissue explants to in vitro compressive overload. Osteoarthritis Cartilage. 2012;20(5):422–9.

116. Dowdy PA, Miniaci A, Arnoczky SP, Fowler PJ, Boughner DR. The effect of cast immobilization on meniscal healing. An experimental study in the dog. Am J Sports Med. 1995;23(6):721–8.

117. Bray RC, Smith JA, Eng MK, Leonard CA, Sutherland CA, Salo PT. Vascular response of the meniscus to injury: effects of immobilization. J Orthop Res. 2001;19(3):384–90.

118. Huang TL, Lin GT, O'Connor S, Chen DY, Barmada R. Healing potential of experimental meniscal tears in the rabbit. Preliminary results. Clin Orthop Relat Res. 1991;267:299–305.

119. Ochi M, Kanda T, Sumen Y, Ikuta Y. Changes in the permeability and histologic findings of rabbit menisci after immobilization. Clin Orthop Relat Res. 1997;334:305–15.

120. Guisasola I, Vaquero J, Forriol F. Knee immobilization on meniscal healing after suture: an experimental

study in sheep. Clin Orthop Relat Res. 2002;395: 227–33.

121. Pavlovich RI. Hi-frequency electrical cautery stimulation in the treatment of displaced meniscal tears. Arthroscopy. 1998;14(6):566–71.

122. Qu F, Esterhai JL, Mauck RL. Modulation of the meniscus repair interface via collagenase delivery from nanofibrous composites. Orthopaedic Research Society annual meeting 2012. Abstract #0776.

123. Zhang H, Leng P, Zhang J. Enhanced meniscal repair by overexpression of hIGF-1 in a full-thickness model. Clin Orthop Relat Res. 2009;467(12):3165–74.

124. Vrancken AC, Buma P, van Tienen TG. Synthetic meniscus replacement: a review. Int Orthop. 2013; 37(2):291–9.

125. Ballyns JJ, Gleghorn JP, Niebrzydowski V, Rawlinson JJ, Potter HG, Maher SA, et al. Image-guided tissue engineering of anatomically shaped implants via MRI and micro-CT using injection molding. Tissue Eng Part A. 2008;14(7): 1195–202.

126. Fisher MB, Henning EA, Soegaard N, Esterhai JL, Mauck RL. Organized nanofibrous scaffolds that mimic the macroscopic and microscopic architecture of the knee meniscus. Acta Biomater. 2013;9(1): 4496–504.

127. Qu F, Lin J, Esterhai JL, Fisher MB, Mauck RL. Improved meniscus integration via controlled degradation of the wound interface. Orthopaedic Research Society annual meeting 2013. Abstract #0562.

Biological Augmentation of Meniscus Repair and Restoration

11

Geoffrey D. Abrams, Joshua D. Harris, Anil K. Gupta, Frank A. McCormick, and Brian J. Cole

Introduction

The meniscus is an important structure for normal knee function. It serves to distribute load, thereby protecting the adjacent articular cartilage, as well as to provide a source of secondary stability for the knee [1, 2]. Meniscal damage can disrupt these critical functions, leading to hyaline cartilage damage and osteoarthritis (OA) (Fig. 11.1) [3]. Because of the association of meniscal damage and the development of OA, attention has been given to the importance of meniscus preservation via repair or replacement.

Healing rates following meniscal repair vary based upon the location of the tear within the knee (medial vs. lateral), location within the meniscus itself (central vs. peripheral), and whether a concomitant anterior cruciate ligament (ACL) reconstruction is being performed. Lateral compartment and peripheral tears with less than 3 mm of rim width are more likely to heal [4]. Successful repairs have been reported to be anywhere from 74 to 96 % when anterior cruciate ligament (ACL) reconstruction is undertaken in the acute injury setting [5, 6]. For isolated meniscal repairs without ACL

reconstruction, however, healing rates are less predictable [7–9]. Most authors speculate the reason for this improved healing following ACL reconstruction is the local delivery of growth and clotting factors from the intra-articular hematoma that develops following femoral and tibial tunnel drilling. In addition, the nature of meniscal injury may differ in the setting of concomitant ACL injury, and meniscal repair may be more successful in this group due to more favorable anatomic tear characteristics. In other words, meniscal tears in conjunction with ACL injury tend to occur more peripherally and usually involve less degenerative tissue.

Given the observation of improved healing rates following concomitant ACL reconstruction and the role of adjunctive growth factors, much attention has been paid to the biologic enhancement of meniscus repairs. Areas of focus have centered on the use of growth factors and cell-based therapies. When repair is not possible, meniscal replacement may be considered. This chapter will review the biology of meniscus healing and use this as a foundation to discuss the enhancement of meniscus repair through mechanical stimulation, growth factors, and gene therapy. It will also discuss current options for meniscal replacement in the meniscus-deficient knee.

G.D. Abrams, M.D. • J.D. Harris, M.D. • A.K. Gupta, M.D., M.B.A. • F.A. McCormick, M.D. • B.J. Cole, M.D., M.B.A. (✉)
Department of Orthopedic Surgery, Rush University Medical Center, 1611 W. Harrison Avenue, Suite 300, Chicago, IL 60612, USA
e-mail: bcole@rushortho.com

Biology of Meniscus Healing

Healing of meniscal repairs is mainly dependent upon tear location as only the outer 10–25 % of the meniscus receives direct blood supply from

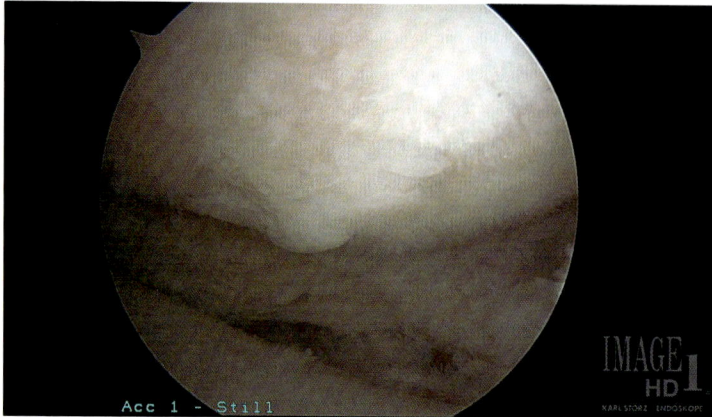

Fig. 11.1 Arthroscopic image demonstrating near full-thickness cartilage loss on the lateral femoral condyle in the knee of a patient with lateral meniscus deficiency. In many cases, meniscus damage is the main factor in cartilage degeneration due to increased stresses on the articular cartilage

the perimeniscal capillary plexus (PCP) [10]. This plexus is supplied by the lateral, medial, and middle geniculate arteries and originates in the capsular and synovial lining of the joint. Nutrient and waste exchange for cells in the inner portion of the meniscus relies on diffusion through the synovial fluid [11]. Blood supply is critical for healing success as the presence of growth and clotting factors simulates the repair process [12–14]. It has been shown that when exposed to these factors, particularly platelet-derived growth factor (PDGF), transforming growth factor-beta (TGF-β), and fibronectin, meniscus fibrochondrocytes are stimulated to proliferate and produce extracellular matrix [15–17].

When a tear occurs in the peripheral portion of the meniscus, a fibrin clot forms which contains inflammatory cells. The PCP then infiltrates the fibrin clot, delivering stem cells and growth factors to aid in the differentiation and growth of the fibrochondrocytes [18, 19]. Some of the growth factors that have been implicated in meniscus healing are PDGF, TGF-β, insulin-like growth factor-1 (IGF-1), vascular endothelial growth factor (VEGF), and basic fibroblast growth factor (bFGF) [19–21]. In an investigation comparing the effect of bFGF, IGF-I, PDGF, and TGF-β on protein and proteoglycan production in bovine meniscus tissue explants, Imler et al. found that all four increased cellular production, with TGF-β being the most potent stimulator [22]. Inflammatory cytokines such as tumor necrosis factor-alpha (TNF-α) and interleukin-1 (IL-1), on the other hand, have been shown to have a deleterious effect on fibrochondrocyte proliferation in vitro [23]. The expression of other molecules, such as the antiangiogenic factor endostatin, also may limit the regeneration capacity of the meniscus [24].

Mechanical Stimulation

Mechanically stimulating the damaged tissue provides an injury response, potentiates vascularity, and is one of the simplest ways to favor healing of the meniscus. The most common techniques utilized are rasping (Fig. 11.2) and trephination. These methods create radially oriented channels to theoretically induce vascular and cellular migration from the periphery to the repair site. Ochi et al. studied the effect of rasping on the presence of TGF-β, PDGF, interleukin-1-alpha (IL-1α), and proliferating cell nuclear antigen (PCNA) on the femoral surface of the menisci following rasping [17]. They found that levels of IL-1α, TGF-β, PDGF, and PCNA on the rasped surface area all reached their peak within 14 days after surgery. Many studies have reported improved healing rates of meniscus tears treated with mechanical stimulation as compared to without [25–27].

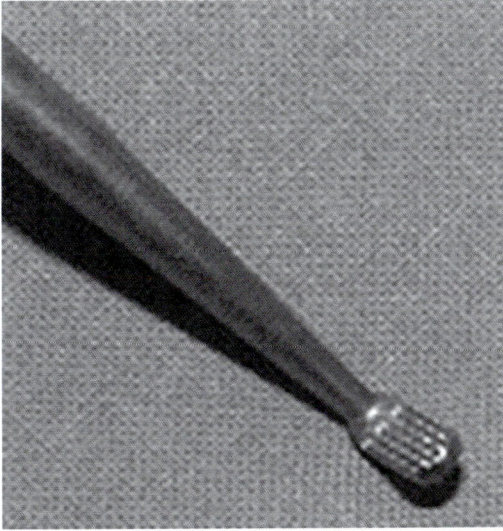

Fig. 11.2 Image of an arthroscopic rasp used for mechanical stimulation of tissue prior to meniscal repair. The rasp is inserted into the meniscal tear in order to improve vascularity at the repair site

Fibrin Clot

Exogenous fibrin clot was one of the first substances studied to aid in the healing of meniscal tears. In 1985 Weber et al. demonstrated that rabbit meniscus fibrochondrocytes proliferate and produce matrix proteins when exposed to the mitogenic factors contained in a wound hematoma [15]. Based upon this initial work, Arnoczky et al. studied the effect of exogenous fibrin clot application on the healing rate of meniscal tears in the avascular region of canines [10]. At 3 and 6 months postoperatively, they reported that all the defects had filled with fibrocartilage-like material. Clinical case series utilizing fibrin clot followed, with van Trommel et al. reporting healing on second look arthroscopy in all patients following repair of peripheral posterior-lateral meniscus tears supplemented with fibrin clot [28]. In a series of 153 meniscus tears with or without concomitant ACL tear, Henning et al. reported a healing rate of 92 % when treated with exogenous fibrin clot versus 59 % for those treated without fibrin, concluding that isolated meniscus tears heal significantly better with the addition of the exogenous agent [29]. In a randomized trial

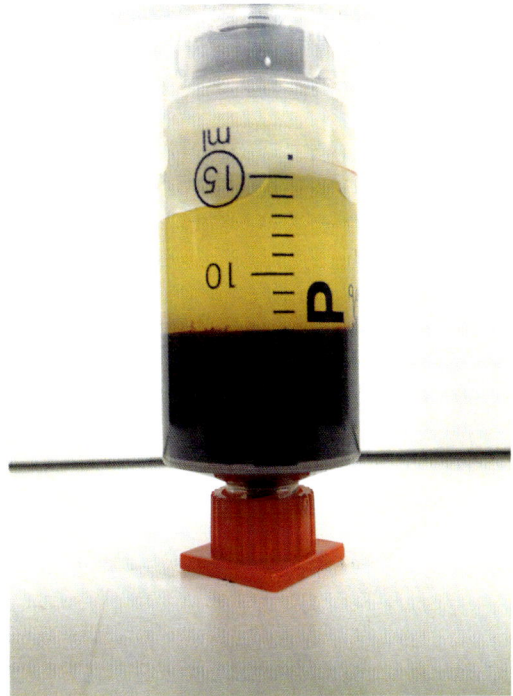

Fig. 11.3 Image showing a syringe with whole blood components following centrifugation. The three layers include the red blood cell base (*bottom*), the buffy coat consisting of platelets and leukocytes (*middle*), and acellular plasma (*top*)

comparing conservative therapy, arthroscopic suture repair with access channels, arthroscopic minimal central resection with intrameniscal fibrin clot and suture repair, and arthroscopic partial meniscectomy, Beidert found 75 %, 90 %, 43 %, and 100 %, respectively, of normal or nearly normal exam and MRI at final follow-up [30]. In other words, the group receiving meniscus repair and fibrin clot application had the lowest clinical and imaging scores. Each group in this study, however, included 12 or fewer patients (with the fibrin clot group consisting of only seven patients), potentially limiting the applicability of this investigation to the larger population.

Platelet-Rich Plasma

Platelet-rich plasma (PRP) is an autologous substance that contains concentrations of platelets above physiologic levels (Fig. 11.3).

These platelets are a source of PDGF, TGF-β, IGF-1, VEGF, and bFGF, among others, and are thought to initiate a healing cascade leading to angiogenesis, matrix production, and cellular proliferation [31–33].

Ishida et al. performed the most comprehensive basic science and animal investigations to date on the effect of PRP on meniscus healing [34]. Using a gelatin hydrogel (GH) to deliver PRP to rabbit meniscal fibrochondrocytes in vitro, they found that levels of growth factors (PDGF, TGF-β, and VEGF) as well as messenger RNA (mRNA) for biglycan and decorin were all higher in cultures supplemented with PRP as compared to platelet-poor plasma (PPP). The authors then used the same delivery system to treat 1.5 mm diameter defects in the avascular zone of rabbit menisci. At 4 weeks, they found residual presence of the hydrogel, indicating elution of the growth factors from PRP took place over this timespan. Histological scoring of the menisci at 12 weeks showed significantly better meniscal healing in the group treated with PRP-infused hydrogel as compared to the hydrogel with PPP or the hydrogel alone [34].

Another investigation examined the effect of hyaluronan-collagen composite matrices without cells, the composite matrices loaded with platelet-rich plasma, autologous bone marrow, or autologous mesenchymal stem cells (MSCs) to treat 2 mm punch defects in the avascular zone of rabbit menisci [35]. At 12 weeks, the authors reported the untreated defects and cell-free composite matrix groups both had a limited fibrocartilaginous healing response. Interestingly, they found that neither the PRP nor bone marrow-loaded matrices showed histological grading improvement as compared to cell-free implants.

Stem Cells

Under the proper conditions, MSCs have the capability of differentiating into a number of different cell lineages and therefore represent a promising option in the augmentation of meniscus repair. There has been documentation of MSCs availability from bone marrow [36] (Fig. 11.4), periosteum [37], adipose tissue [38], and the synovial lining

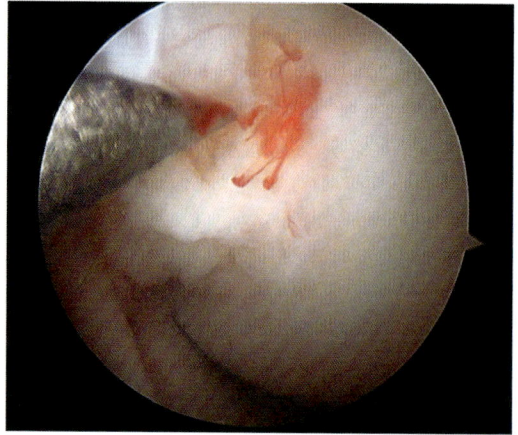

Fig. 11.4 Arthroscopic image showing microfracture of the wall of medial femoral condyle within the notch. This technique allows for mesenchymal stem cells (MSC) within the bone marrow to have access to the meniscus itself and augment healing

of major joints [39]. In both cartilage and meniscus restoration investigations, they are commonly delivered to the desired treatment area through the use of a cellular scaffold [40, 41].

Bone Marrow-Derived Stem Cells

Using autologous-derived bone marrow MSCs in a rabbit meniscus defect model, Zellner et al. studied the effect of a precultured chondrogenic MSC matrix construct versus non-precultured stem cell-matrices [35]. Preculturing of the MSCs took place in a chondrogenic medium and MSCs were implanted in a hyaluronan-ester and gelatin scaffold. They found that the precultured cells lead to fibrocartilage-like repair tissue and had only partial integration with the native meniscus. On the other hand, non-precultured MSC matrices demonstrated more complete fill and meniscus-like healing on histological sectioning [35]. Other investigations utilizing different animal models and a variety of scaffolds have shown promising results with the use of bone marrow-derived MSCs [42–44].

Yet another way to allow MSC delivery to the meniscus in order to augment healing is with the use of microfracture [45]. In their article, Freedman et al. describe the use of microfracture following standard techniques for mechanical stimulation and then inside-out meniscus repair, although the microfracture technique can be utilized following any meniscus repair method. Following repair, a 45° microfracture awl is placed through the contralateral portal. The awl is repeatedly penetrated through the subchondral bone of the intercondylar notch at the posterior cruciate ligament (PCL) origin until marrow elements are seen to enter the joint. The flow of arthroscopic fluid can be halted to more accurately confirm blood flow emanating from the microfracture sites [45].

Synovial-Derived Stem Cells

Many investigators advocate for the use of synovial-derived MSCs as they can be easily harvested and have shown the ability to easily expand in culture [46]. Using autologous MSCs harvested from rabbits, Horie et al. studied regenerative efforts after cylindrical defects were created in the avascular portion of the medial meniscus [47]. During the index procedure, the defect was created through an open arthrotomy in each knee. One knee received a direct injection of suspended MSCs, while the other received only an injection of phosphate buffered saline (PBS) as a control. They found that the quantity of the regenerative tissue was greater at all timepoints for the MSC group, reaching significance at the 4- and 12-week marks, while the quality of the regenerative was also significantly higher at 12 and 24 weeks. Another investigation which injected synovial-derived MSCs into the knees of meniscectomized rats found improved adherence to the defect site, differentiation into meniscal cells, and promotion of meniscus regeneration in the MSC group as compared to controls [47].

Adipose-Derived Stem Cells (ADSC)

Yet another source of MSCs is from adipose tissue. Ruiz-Iban used ADSCs to investigate meniscus healing potentiation in a rabbit model [48]. Using the contralateral knee as a control, they injected labeled MSCs directly into the tear after either immediately repairing the lesion with suture or after performing the repair 3 weeks later. Results showed that the addition of ADSCs to the repair site significantly increased the healing rate with the repair sites showing well-formed meniscal fibrocartilage made up of cells which had differentiated from the previously injected ADSCs.

Meniscus Replacement

Meniscus repair is not always possible, particularly in the case of complex tears. Debridement of large tears may lead to meniscal deficiency after debridement. In young patients who are not candidates for arthroplasty, meniscus replacement is an option. Choices for replacement include allograft transplantation, collagen-based scaffolds, and synthetic scaffolds.

Allograft Transplantation

In contrast to collagen-based and synthetic scaffolds, meniscus allograft transplantation can be used in cases of complete meniscus deficiency (Fig. 11.5a, b). The procedure has shown good results at mid- and long-term follow-up. In a study of patients undergoing both isolated transplant and combined procedures, Saltzman et al. reported significant improvement in all functional scores as well as an average overall satisfaction of 8.8 out of 10 [49]. Overall success rate at a minimum of 7-year follow-up was 88 %. Another investigation of meniscus transplantation with or without high tibial osteotomy (HTO) with a minimum 10-year follow-up reported a significantly improved modified Hospital for Special Surgery (HSS) score for all groups [50]. Those undergoing combined medial meniscus transplantation (MMT) and HTO showed greater functional improvement compared to MMT alone. There was no progression of radiographic changes in 41 % of knees and no further changes in cartilage signal on MRI in 36 %. In combination with articular cartilage repair or restoration, meniscus transplantation only has a reported

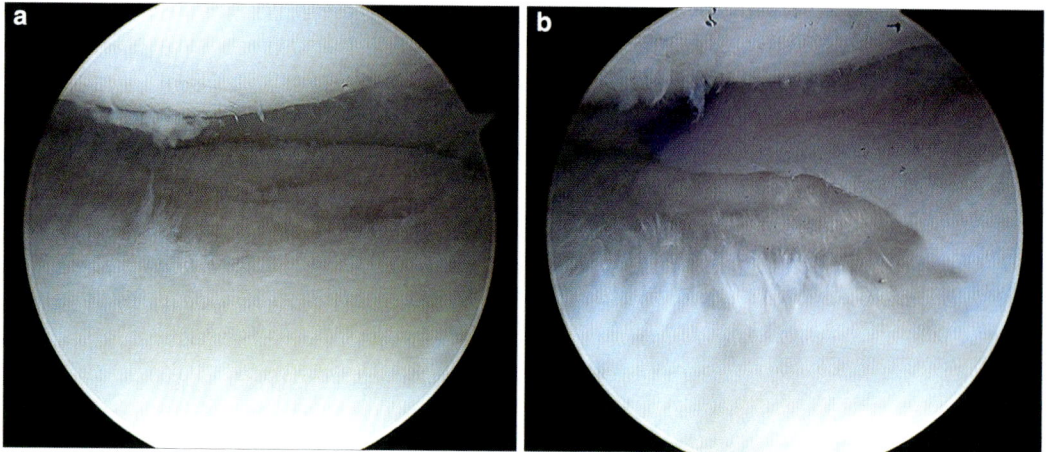

Fig. 11.5 (**a**) Arthroscopic image showing a near complete meniscectomized state in the medial compartment of a 24-year-old female. (**b**) Same compartment following meniscus transplantation with a size-matched allograft using bone block fixation

12 % failure rate [51]. Rue et al. reported on patients undergoing meniscus transplantation in combination with either autologous chondrocyte implantation (ACI) or osteochondral allograft (OA). At a minimum of 2-year follow-up, 76 % of participants reported satisfaction with their clinical results and 90 % of participants would have the surgery again [52]. A number of other studies have supported the use of transplantation for those with meniscus deficiency [53–55].

Collagen-Based and Synthetic Menisci

Unlike allograft meniscus transplantation, use of collagen or synthetically manufactured menisci requires an intact anterior and posterior horn as well as a small peripheral rim where the meniscus can be attached. Manaflex® or collagen meniscus implant/CMI (ReGen Biologics, Hackensack, NJ, USA) is an artificial meniscus derived from bovine collagen which is not currently approved for use in the United States. An initial report on eight patients showed promising results at short-term follow-up [56]. This was followed by a multicenter, randomized clinical trial comparing the use of the implant versus meniscectomy in over 300 patients with acute and chronic meniscal deficiency [57]. With a mean duration of follow-up of 59 months, the authors reported that in the chronic group, patients that had received the implant regained more of their lost ability as compared to the control meniscectomy group. There were no statistically significant differences in functional outcome in the acute replacement group.

Synthetic meniscus scaffolds have also been investigated. Actifit® (Orteq Bioengineering, London, UK) is a biodegradable polyurethane scaffold designed for meniscus replacement. In a recently published case series, 52 patients with irreparable meniscal defects were implanted with the synthetic scaffold [58]. Statistically significant improvement in International Knee Documentation Committee (IKDC), Knee Injury and Osteoarthritis Outcome Score (KOOS), and Lysholm scores was seen at 2-year follow-up as compared to preoperatively. Overall treatment failure rate was 17 % and there were nine implant related serious adverse events requiring reoperation.

Enzymatic Inhibition

Increased levels of inflammatory cytokines are associated with injuries to the knee. These inflammatory cytokines increase enzymatic tissue degradation and suppress matrix biosynthesis [59]. Investigations have demonstrated that IL-1 dose dependently decreases the shear strength of meniscus repair through inhibition of tissue formation at the meniscus repair interface [60–62]. Hennerbichler et al. harvested cylindrical explants from the outer one-third of the medial meniscus in a porcine model. The explants were immediately replaced and the entire specimen was incubated in medium with and without recombinant porcine IL-1. Those cultured in medium with IL-1 showed no discernable repair tissue despite the presence of viable cells [62]. The mechanism through which IL-1 provides its detrimental effects to meniscus healing is not fully understood. Recent evidence, however, has shown that matrix metalloproteinases (MMP) may play a role. McNulty et al. demonstrated that even in the presence of IL-1, a broad-spectrum MMP inhibitor increased the shear strength of meniscus repair sites and enhanced tissue repair at the interface compared to samples without MMP inhibitor [63]. Given these data, the search is underway for the optimal cytokine and/or MMP inhibitor in the attempt to enhance meniscus healing rates.

Genetic Modification

An investigational method of meniscal regeneration involves virus-mediated transfer of a growth factor's complementary deoxyribonucleic acid (cDNA) into stem cells [64]. The studies which have been published in this area have demonstrated the feasibility of direct delivery of TGF-β1 cDNA into meniscal tissue [65, 66]. Goto et al. investigated the use of genetically modified bovine meniscal cells and MSCs cultured in a collagen-glycosaminoglycan (GAG) matrix [67]. They showed that after 3 weeks of in vitro culture, transfer of TGF-β1 cDNA into the cells increased cell density and also the synthesis of proteoglycans and type-II collagen. Furthermore, transplantation of the transduced constructs into the avascular zone of bovine meniscal lesions resulted in filling of the lesions with repair tissue. The authors concluded that growth factor delivery through cDNA transduction may provide potentiation for meniscal healing and repair.

Senior Author's Preferred Treatment Method

Meniscus preservation and repair is preferred to meniscectomy when possible, particularly in the young patient. For small meniscus tears that are amenable to repair, an all-inside technique is used. For larger tears, such as bucket-handle type tears, standard inside-out technique with alternating vertical mattress sutures is performed. To augment healing following repair, microfracture within the intercondylar notch (Fig. 11.4) is most commonly carried out to potentially allow MSCs to access the repair site. In addition, PRP is occasionally injected into the joint following repair.

Case Presentation

Figure 11.6a demonstrates a bucket-handle type tear of the lateral meniscus in the left knee of a 17-year-old football player who sustained a twisting injury to the knee. Preoperative exam and imaging were consistent with an isolated tear of the lateral meniscus. Intraoperative exam under anesthesia confirmed a negative pivot shift and arthroscopic evaluation of the anterior cruciate ligament showed it to be intact. Because of the large area of involved meniscus and the young age of the patient, meniscus repair was undertaken using standard inside-out repair technique (Fig. 11.6b). Following the repair, meniscus healing was augmented with microfracture of the intercondylar notch area to provide the repair milieu with autogeneic MSCs.

Conclusion

Meniscus preservation via repair or allograft transplantation should be the goal of any surgeon treating meniscus pathology. Meniscus repair, when possible, remains the optimum treatment for meniscus tears. Augmentation of the repair process using a variety of techniques and substances has been investigated, but other than mechanical stimulation at the time of repair, none

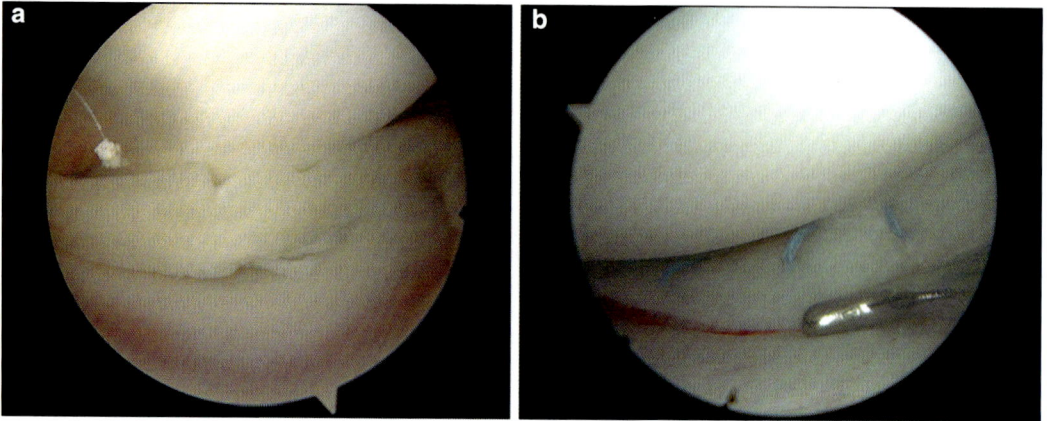

Fig. 11.6 (**a**, **b**) Arthroscopic image from the anterolateral portal demonstrating a bucket-handle type tear in the peripheral zone of the lateral meniscus (**a**) prior to and (**b**) following repair with inside-out meniscus repair technique. This repair was subsequently augmented with microfracture of the intercondylar notch

has gained widespread use. In the case of meniscal deficiency, allograft transplantation remains the most commonly performed procedure. Collagen and synthetic meniscal implants, as well as utilization of growth factors and stem cells, remain investigational.

References

1. Bedi A, Kelly NH, Baad M, et al. Dynamic contact mechanics of the medial meniscus as a function of radial tear, repair, and partial meniscectomy. J Bone Joint Surg Am. 2010;92:1398–408.
2. Ahn JH, Bae TS, Kang KS, et al. Longitudinal tear of the medial meniscus posterior horn in the anterior cruciate ligament-deficient knee significantly influences anterior stability. Am J Sports Med. 2011;39:2187–93.
3. Bonneux I, Vandekerckhove B. Arthroscopic partial lateral meniscectomy long-term results in athletes. Acta Orthop Belg. 2002;68:356–61.
4. Greis PE, Holmstrom MC, Bardana DD, et al. Meniscal injury: II. Management. J Am Acad Orthop Surg. 2002;10:177–87.
5. Toman CV, Dunn WR, Spindler KP, et al. Success of meniscal repair at anterior cruciate ligament reconstruction. Am J Sports Med. 2009;37:1111–5.
6. Tachibana Y, Sakaguchi K, Goto T, et al. Repair integrity evaluated by second-look arthroscopy after arthroscopic meniscal repair with the FasT-Fix during anterior cruciate ligament reconstruction. Am J Sports Med. 2010;38:965–71.
7. Logan M, Watts M, Owen J, et al. Meniscal repair in the elite athlete: results of 45 repairs with a minimum 5-year follow-up. Am J Sports Med. 2009;37:1131–4.
8. Majewski M, Stoll R, Widmer H, et al. Midterm and long-term results after arthroscopic suture repair of isolated, longitudinal, vertical meniscal tears in stable knees. Am J Sports Med. 2006;34:1072–6.
9. Haas AL, Schepsis AA, Hornstein J, et al. Meniscal repair using the FasT-Fix all-inside meniscal repair device. Arthroscopy. 2005;21:167–75.
10. Arnoczky SP, Warren RF. Microvasculature of the human meniscus. Am J Sports Med. 1982;10:90–5.
11. Gershuni DH, Hargens AR, Danzig LA. Regional nutrition and cellularity of the meniscus. Implications for tear and repair. Sports Med. 1988;5:322–7.
12. Lee SY, Niikura T, Reddi AH. Superficial zone protein (lubricin) in the different tissue compartments of the knee joint: modulation by transforming growth factor beta 1 and interleukin-1 beta. Tissue Eng Part A. 2008;14:1799–808.
13. Bhargava MM, Hidaka C, Hannafin JA, et al. Effects of hepatocyte growth factor and platelet-derived growth factor on the repair of meniscal defects in vitro. In Vitro Cell Dev Biol Anim. 2005;41:305–10.
14. Kamimura T, Kimura M. Repair of horizontal meniscal cleavage tears with exogenous fibrin clots. Knee Surg Sports Traumatol Arthrosc. 2011;19:1154–7.
15. Webber RJ, Harris MG, Hough Jr AJ. Cell culture of rabbit meniscal fibrochondrocytes: proliferative and synthetic response to growth factors and ascorbate. J Orthop Res. 1985;3:36–42.
16. Tumia NS, Johnstone AJ. Platelet derived growth factor-AB enhances knee meniscal cell activity in vitro. Knee. 2009;16:73–6.
17. Ochi M, Uchio Y, Okuda K, et al. Expression of cytokines after meniscal rasping to promote meniscal healing. Arthroscopy. 2001;17:724–31.
18. Nakata K, Shino K, Hamada M, et al. Human meniscus cell: characterization of the primary culture and use for tissue engineering. Clin Orthop Relat Res. 2001:S208–18.

19. Scordino LE, Deberardino TM. Biologic enhancement of meniscus repair. Clin Sports Med. 2012;31:91–100.

20. Petersen W, Pufe T, Starke C, et al. Locally applied angiogenic factors—a new therapeutic tool for meniscal repair. Ann Anat. 2005;187:509–19.

21. Makris EA, Hadidi P, Athanasiou KA. The knee meniscus: structure–function, pathophysiology, current repair techniques, and prospects for regeneration. Biomaterials. 2011;32:7411–31.

22. Imler SM, Doshi AN, Levenston ME. Combined effects of growth factors and static mechanical compression on meniscus explant biosynthesis. Osteoarthritis Cartilage. 2004;12:736–44.

23. Riera KM, Rothfusz NE, Wilusz RE, et al. Interleukin-1, tumor necrosis factor-alpha, and transforming growth factor-beta 1 and integrative meniscal repair: influences on meniscal cell proliferation and migration. Arthritis Res Ther. 2011;13:R187.

24. Hoberg M, Schmidt EL, Tuerk M, et al. Induction of endostatin expression in meniscal fibrochondrocytes by co-culture with endothelial cells. Arch Orthop Trauma Surg. 2009;129:1137–43.

25. Zhang Z, Arnold JA, Williams T, et al. Repairs by trephination and suturing of longitudinal injuries in the avascular area of the meniscus in goats. Am J Sports Med. 1995;23:35–41.

26. Uchio Y, Ochi M, Adachi N, et al. Results of rasping of meniscal tears with and without anterior cruciate ligament injury as evaluated by second-look arthroscopy. Arthroscopy. 2003;19:463–9.

27. Henning CE, Lynch MA, Clark JR. Vascularity for healing of meniscus repairs. Arthroscopy. 1987;3:13–8.

28. van Trommel MF, Simonian PT, Potter HG, et al. Arthroscopic meniscal repair with fibrin clot of complete radial tears of the lateral meniscus in the avascular zone. Arthroscopy. 1998;14:360–5.

29. Henning CE, Lynch MA, Yearout KM, et al. Arthroscopic meniscal repair using an exogenous fibrin clot. Clin Orthop Relat Res. 1990:64–72.

30. Biedert RM. Treatment of intrasubstance meniscal lesions: a randomized prospective study of four different methods. Knee Surg Sports Traumatol Arthrosc. 2000;8:104–8.

31. Foster TE, Puskas BL, Mandelbaum BR, et al. Platelet-rich plasma: from basic science to clinical applications. Am J Sports Med. 2009;37:2259–72.

32. Eppley BL, Woodell JE, Higgins J. Platelet quantification and growth factor analysis from platelet-rich plasma: implications for wound healing. Plast Reconstr Surg. 2004;114:1502–8.

33. Delos D, Rodeo SA. Enhancing meniscal repair through biology: platelet-rich plasma as an alternative strategy. Instr Course Lect. 2011;60:453–60.

34. Ishida K, Kuroda R, Miwa M, et al. The regenerative effects of platelet-rich plasma on meniscal cells in vitro and its in vivo application with biodegradable gelatin hydrogel. Tissue Eng. 2007;13:1103–12.

35. Zellner J, Mueller M, Berner A, et al. Role of mesenchymal stem cells in tissue engineering of meniscus. J Biomed Mater Res A. 2010;94:1150–61.

36. Prockop DJ. Marrow stromal cells as stem cells for nonhematopoietic tissues. Science. 1997;276:71–4.

37. De Bari C, Dell'Accio F, Vanlauwe J, et al. Mesenchymal multipotency of adult human periosteal cells demonstrated by single-cell lineage analysis. Arthritis Rheum. 2006;54:1209–21.

38. Zuk PA, Zhu M, Ashjian P, et al. Human adipose tissue is a source of multipotent stem cells. Mol Biol Cell. 2002;13:4279–95.

39. De Bari C, Dell'Accio F, Tylzanowski P, et al. Multipotent mesenchymal stem cells from adult human synovial membrane. Arthritis Rheum. 2001;44:1928–42.

40. Gu Y, Zhu W, Hao Y, et al. Repair of meniscal defect using an induced myoblast-loaded polyglycolic acid mesh in a canine model. Exp Ther Med. 2012;3:293–8.

41. Maher SA, Rodeo SA, Potter HG, et al. A pre-clinical test platform for the functional evaluation of scaffolds for musculoskeletal defects: the meniscus. HSS J. 2011;7:157–63.

42. Pabbruwe MB, Kafienah W, Tarlton JF, et al. Repair of meniscal cartilage white zone tears using a stem cell/collagen-scaffold implant. Biomaterials. 2010;31:2583–91.

43. Izuta Y, Ochi M, Adachi N, et al. Meniscal repair using bone marrow-derived mesenchymal stem cells: experimental study using green fluorescent protein transgenic rats. Knee. 2005;12:217–23.

44. Angele P, Johnstone B, Kujat R, et al. Stem cell based tissue engineering for meniscus repair. J Biomed Mater Res A. 2008;85:445–55.

45. Freedman KB, Nho SJ, Cole BJ. Marrow stimulating technique to augment meniscus repair. Arthroscopy. 2003;19:794–8.

46. Yoshimura H, Muneta T, Nimura A, et al. Comparison of rat mesenchymal stem cells derived from bone marrow, synovium, periosteum, adipose tissue, and muscle. Cell Tissue Res. 2007;327:449–62.

47. Horie M, Driscoll MD, Sampson HW, et al. Implantation of allogenic synovial stem cells promotes meniscal regeneration in a rabbit meniscal defect model. J Bone Joint Surg Am. 2012;94:701–12.

48. Ruiz-Iban MA, Diaz-Heredia J, Garcia-Gomez I, et al. The effect of the addition of adipose-derived mesenchymal stem cells to a meniscal repair in the avascular zone: an experimental study in rabbits. Arthroscopy. 2011;27:1688–96.

49. Saltzman BM, Bajaj S, Salata M, et al. Prospective long-term evaluation of meniscal allograft transplantation procedure: a minimum of 7-year follow-up. J Knee Surg. 2012;25:165–75.

50. Verdonk PC, Verstraete KL, Almqvist KF, et al. Meniscal allograft transplantation: long-term clinical results with radiological and magnetic resonance imaging correlations. Knee Surg Sports Traumatol Arthrosc. 2006;14:694–706.

51. Harris JD, Cavo M, Brophy R, et al. Biological knee reconstruction: a systematic review of combined meniscal allograft transplantation and cartilage repair or restoration. Arthroscopy. 2011;27:409–18.

52. Rue JP, Yanke AB, Busam ML, et al. Prospective evaluation of concurrent meniscus transplantation and articular cartilage repair: minimum 2-year follow-up. Am J Sports Med. 2008;36:1770–8.

53. van der Wal RJ, Thomassen BJ, van Arkel ER. Long-term clinical outcome of open meniscal allograft transplantation. Am J Sports Med. 2009;37:2134–9.

54. Marcacci M, Zaffagnini S, Marcheggiani Muccioli GM, et al. Meniscal allograft transplantation without bone plugs: a 3-year minimum follow-up study. Am J Sports Med. 2012;40:395–403.

55. Kim JM, Lee BS, Kim KH, et al. Results of meniscus allograft transplantation using bone fixation: 110 cases with objective evaluation. Am J Sports Med. 2012;40:1027–34.

56. Rodkey WG, Steadman JR, Li ST. A clinical study of collagen meniscus implants to restore the injured meniscus. Clin Orthop Relat Res. 1999:S281–92.

57. Rodkey WG, DeHaven KE, Montgomery III WH, et al. Comparison of the collagen meniscus implant with partial meniscectomy. A prospective randomized trial. J Bone Joint Surg Am. 2008;90:1413–26.

58. Verdonk P, Beaufils P, Bellemans J, et al. Successful treatment of painful irreparable partial meniscal defects with a polyurethane scaffold: two-year safety and clinical outcomes. Am J Sports Med. 2012;40:844–53.

59. Hopkins SJ, Humphreys M, Jayson MI. Cytokines in synovial fluid. I. The presence of biologically active and immunoreactive IL-1. Clin Exp Immunol. 1988;72:422–7.

60. Ferretti M, Madhavan S, Deschner J, et al. Dynamic biophysical strain modulates proinflammatory gene induction in meniscal fibrochondrocytes. Am J Physiol Cell Physiol. 2006;290:C1610–5.

61. Wilusz RE, Weinberg JB, Guilak F, et al. Inhibition of integrative repair of the meniscus following acute exposure to interleukin-1 in vitro. J Orthop Res. 2008;26:504–12.

62. Hennerbichler A, Moutos FT, Hennerbichler D, et al. Interleukin-1 and tumor necrosis factor alpha inhibit repair of the porcine meniscus in vitro. Osteoarthritis Cartilage. 2007;15:1053–60.

63. McNulty AL, Weinberg JB, Guilak F. Inhibition of matrix metalloproteinases enhances in vitro repair of the meniscus. Clin Orthop Relat Res. 2009;467:1557–67.

64. Evans CH, Robbins PD. Genetically augmented tissue engineering of the musculoskeletal system. Clin Orthop Relat Res. 1999:S410–8.

65. Goto H, Shuler FD, Niyibizi C, et al. Gene therapy for meniscal injury: enhanced synthesis of proteoglycan and collagen by meniscal cells transduced with a TGFbeta(1)gene. Osteoarthritis Cartilage. 2000;8:266–71.

66. Goto H, Shuler FD, Lamsam C, et al. Transfer of lacZ marker gene to the meniscus. J Bone Joint Surg Am. 1999;81:918–25.

67. Steinert AF, Palmer GD, Capito R, et al. Genetically enhanced engineering of meniscus tissue using ex vivo delivery of transforming growth factor-beta 1 complementary deoxyribonucleic acid. Tissue Eng. 2007;13:2227–37.

Rehabilitation Following Meniscus Repair

Brian Eckenrode and Marisa Pontillo

Introduction and General Rehabilitation Principles

Rehabilitation of patients following meniscus repair requires a thorough understanding of the anatomy and biomechanics of the lower extremity in addition to knowledge of the procedure and patient-specific lesion pathology. The guidelines presented here are designed towards patients with an isolated meniscus repair and should be modified to consider any concomitant injuries or surgeries. The goal of this rehabilitation protocol is to maximize function for a successful outcome and prevent future degeneration while minimizing potentially harmful forces and promoting healing of the repaired tissue.

Postoperatively, physical therapists should consider the type, location, and size of the meniscus tear. These factors will alter the time frames for weight-bearing and necessitate knee range of motion (ROM) limitations during exercise. Repairs to the periphery of the meniscus heal rapidly due to a greater vascular supply, while complex and more central repairs heal slowly and require prolonged protection from adverse forces [1].

B. Eckenrode, P.T., D.P.T., O.C.S. (✉)
Department of Physical Therapy, Arcadia University,
Glenside, PA, USA
e-mail: eckenrodeb@arcadia.edu

M. Pontillo, P.T., D.P.T., S.C.S.
GSPP Penn Therapy and Fitness at Penn Sports
Medicine Center, Philadelphia, PA, USA

Weight-bearing limitations are designed to control the high compressive and shear forces that could disrupt the healing meniscus in the early phases of rehabilitation [1]. For patients with a radial repair, excessive weight-bearing early after surgery can disrupt the repair site [1]. As stated, peripheral meniscal repairs heal more rapidly, whereas complex multiplanar repairs, which extend into the central one-third of the meniscus, tend to heal more slowly [2]. The amount of cartilage degeneration is also an important factor to consider during the postoperative course and should be determined via physician communication or from the operative report.

The postoperative physical therapy of a meniscus repair can be divided into early (immediate postoperative and subacute) and late rehabilitation phases (functional progression and return to sport or occupation). Similar to other postoperative protocols (e.g., anterior cruciate ligament reconstruction), specific goals and time from surgery are used as determinants for phase progression. Recently, a greater emphasis has been placed on criteria-based progressions, which allow the patient to progress at a more individualized pace while simultaneously respecting healing tissues. Notably, the phases below have approximate time guidelines, but the patient must also meet the stated criteria goals prior to moving on to the subsequent phase. The postoperative rehabilitation of patients following repair of the meniscus will be discussed here and is outlined in Table 12.1. During the course of rehabilitation, the therapist should constantly monitor knee joint

Table 12.1 Meniscus repair postoperative protocol [1]

Phase 1: Postop phase	
Goals	

- Protect healing of repair
- Decrease pain
- Manage effusion
- Increase weight-bearing tolerance per procedure
- Gradually improve knee ROM to 0–90° by week 2 and 0–120° by week 4
- Restore quadriceps control

Weeks 1–2	
Brace	Long-leg postoperative brace
ROM goals	0–90°
Weight bearing	Peripheral. TTWB – 50 % WB
	Complex: TTWB – 25 % WB
Interventions	Patella mobilizations
	LE flexibility
	Quad set/SLR/knee extension AROM
	NMES
	Ankle pumps
	Ice/compression/elevation

Weeks 3–4	
Brace	Long-leg postoperative brace
ROM goals	0–120°
Weight-bearing	Peripheral, 75 % FWB; complex, 50–75 % WB
Interventions	Patella mobilizations
	LE flexibility
	Quad set/SLR/knee extension AROM
	NMES
	Ankle pumps
	HR/wall sits (peripheral)
	Ice/compression/elevation

Phase 2: Early rehab phase	
Goals	

- Gradually improve knee ROM to full
- Minimal to no effusion
- Decrease pain
- Progress weight-bearing tolerance per procedure
- Increase strength
- Improve balance and proprioception
- Minimal to no gait deviations

Weeks 5–6	
Brace	Long-leg postoperative brace
ROM goals	0–135°
Weight-bearing	Peripheral, FWB; Complex, 75 % FWB
Interventions	Patella mobilizations
	LE flexibility
	Quad set/SLR
	NMES
	Knee extension 90–30°
	Leg press 70–10° (peripheral)
	Mini squats/HR/wall sits
	Ice/compression/elevation

(continued)

Table 12.1 (continued)

Phase 2: Early rehab phase	
Weeks 7–8	
ROM goals	Full ROM
Weight-bearing	FWB
Interventions	LE flexibility
	Quad set/SLR
	Knee extension 90–30°
	Multi-hip (Flex/ABD/ADD/Ext)
	Ham curls
	Leg press 70–10° (peripheral)
	Mini squats/HR/wall sits
	Lateral step-ups
	Proprioception
	Stationary bike
	Ice/compression/elevation

Phase 3: Functional progression	
Goals	

- Improve lower extremity strength
- Enhance proprioception, balance, and neuromuscular control
- Improve muscular endurance
- Restore limb confidence and function

Weeks 9–12+	
Interventions	LE flexibility
	Quad set/SLR
	Knee extension 90–30°
	Multi-hip (Flex/ABD/ADD/Ext)
	Ham curls
	Leg press 70–10°
	Mini squats/HR/wall sits
	Lunges
	Sports cord/band walks
	Proprioception
	Perturbation training
	Stationary bike
	Swimming
	Stair climber
	Ice/compression/elevation

Phase 4: Return to activity	

- Normalize lower extremity strength
- Enhance muscular power and endurance
- Improve neuromuscular control
- Completion of running program
- Perform selected sport-specific drills
- Gradual return to full unrestricted sports

4–6+ months	
Interventions	LE flexibility
	Knee extension 90–30°
	Multi-hip (Flex/ABD/ADD/Ext)
	Ham curls
	Leg press 70–10°
	Mini squats/HR/wall sits

(continued)

Table 12.1 (continued)

Phase 4: Return to activity
        Proprioception
        Stationary bike
        Swimming
        Stair climber
        Running program
          4 months peripheral
          6 months complex
        Plyometrics (peripheral tears
        4–6 months/complex tears
        6–9 months)

effusion, pain, gait, knee ROM, patella mobility, strength, and flexibility and for any joint-related symptoms indicative of a meniscus tear [2]. The importance of a home exercise program in conjunction with physical therapy is vital for a successful outcome.

Phase 1: Postoperative (Weeks 1–4)

The immediate postoperative phase begins following surgery and lasts approximately 1 month. Initially, patients ambulate with bilateral axillary crutches in a postoperative long-leg brace locked in full extension. Limited weight-bearing for the first 4 weeks may protect the repair and increase the healing potential. Generally, for a peripheral repair, patients will be toe-touch weight-bearing to 50 % weight-bearing during this time interval. For complex and radial tears, patients will be toe-touch weight-bearing to 25 % weight-bearing. For radial tears, it has been reported that weight-bearing may place a displacing force across the repair of a radial meniscus tear; thus weight-bearing precautions will be similar to a complex tear [3]. However, early physiological loading can be beneficial to the menisci in a manner similar to fractures and may help overall healing [4]. The knee brace is opened from 0° to 90° for ROM exercises and kept locked in extension for all other activities. Flexion beyond 90° is discouraged for the first month since motion beyond this leads to "femoral rollback" and therefore increased tensile forces across the repair site. Ice, compression, and elevation are important for

controlling knee effusion and pain control. Patients are instructed to utilize ice for 10–15 min every 1–2 h during the first 10–14 days postoperatively.

Formal physical therapy is initiated within the first 2 weeks postoperatively. Knee ROM exercises are initiated at this time, with the goal of providing a controlled passive tissue stretch while minimizing pain and reactivity. The surgeon may also recommend use of a continuous passive motion machine (CPM) to aid in regaining range of motion with minimal stress on the healing tissues. Two exercises to address knee flexion ROM are supine passive heel slides and wall slides (Fig. 12.1). These exercises are held for 10–15 s, 5–10 repetitions, 3–5 times per day. The importance of early knee range of motion may prevent meniscal atrophy and decreased collagen content [3]. The goal for knee flexion ROM would be to achieve 90° by 2 weeks and 120° by 4 weeks. The authors recommend avoiding active knee flexion during this phase to minimize hamstring strain to the posteromedial knee joint. Manual techniques of gentle passive knee flexion ROM and patella mobilizations are also indicated in this phase.

Achieving full passive knee extension is vital to a normal gait and to minimize additional complications. Furthermore, repaired longitudinal tears of the menisci realize the least strain across the anastomosis when the knee is in full extension. Heel props and prone hangs can be implemented to achieve full passive knee extension ROM (Fig. 12.2). These can be performed for 5–10 min every 1–2 h. Hamstring and gastroc–soleus complex stretching in non-weight-bearing can also be initiated. For patients who underwent an anterior horn repair, knee hyperextension should be avoided.

Patients should be able to perform an active quadriceps contraction with the knee in extension with a visible and palpable superior glide of the patella. This isometric quadriceps setting may be enhanced through the use of neuromuscular electric stimulation (NMES). The benefit of NMES is that it directly recruits the motor neurons to produce improved quadriceps strength gains than

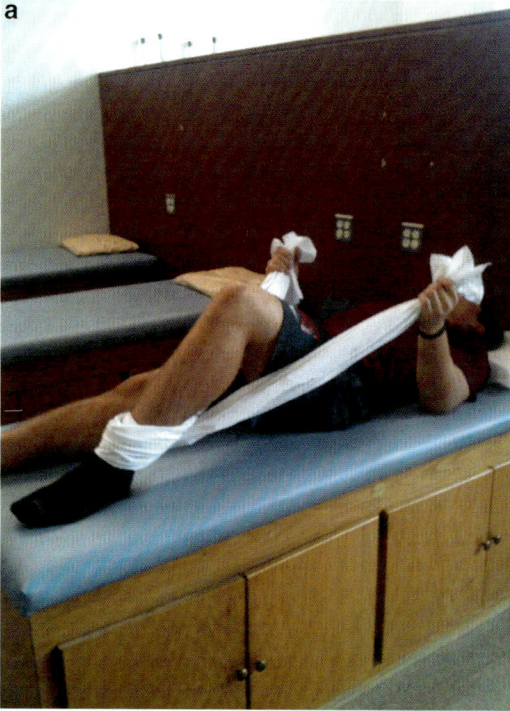

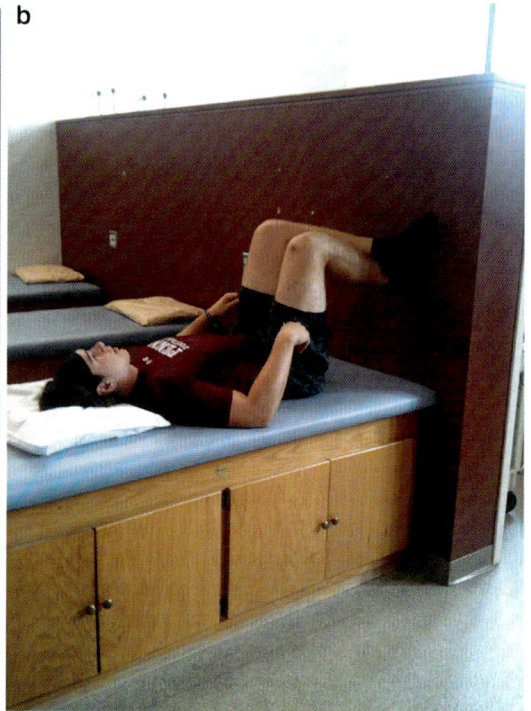

Fig. 12.1 Supine passive heel slides (**a**) and wall slides (**b**) are designed to passively increase knee flexion range of motion based upon the stage of rehabilitation. Active activation of the hamstrings is minimized in both exercises

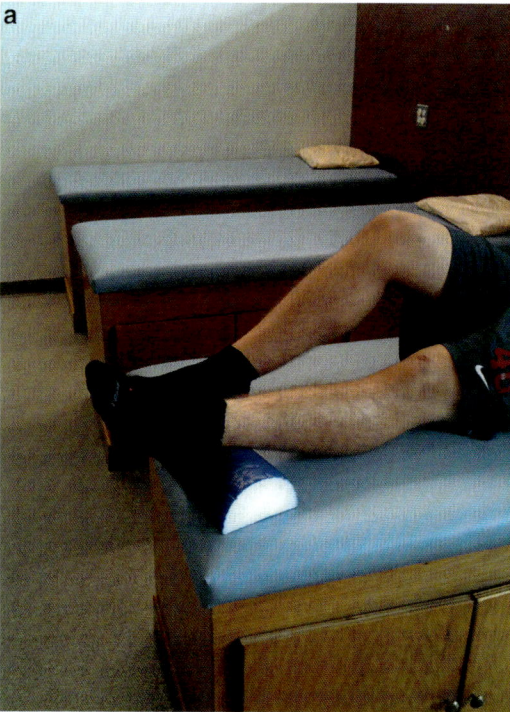

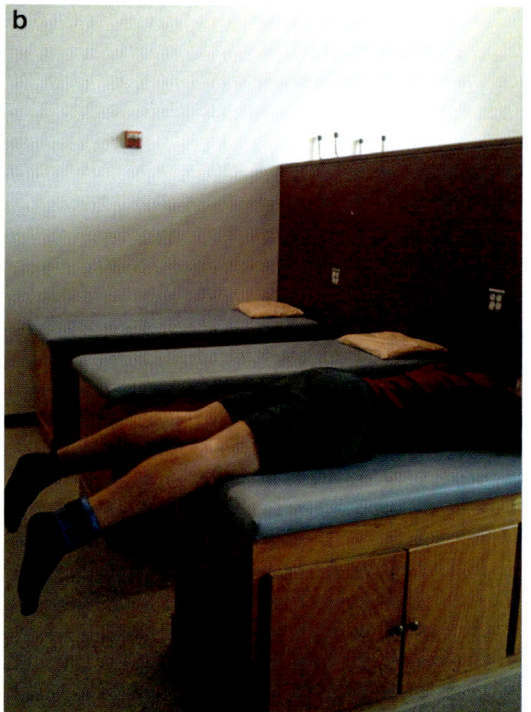

Fig. 12.2 Heel props (**a**) and prone hangs (**b**) are key exercises to address passive knee extension range of motion (ROM). A low-load, long-duration stretch is applied during these exercises to cause tissue elongation with the goal of achieving symmetrical extension (ROM) as compared to the uninvolved knee. With the prone hang (**b**), the patella is positioned so that it lies off of the plinth, and the patient is instructed to maintain the hips on the surface to prevent rotational compensation proximally. A cuff weight can be added at the ankle to create over-pressure into extension range of motion

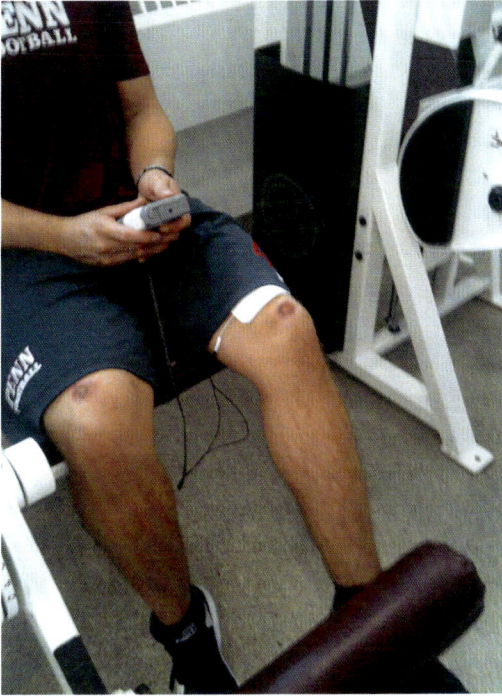

Fig. 12.3 The suggested application of NMES to the involved quadriceps is with the patient seated with the knee in approximately 60° of flexion

voluntary exercise alone [5]. Electrodes for application of the NMES are placed over the proximal lateral quadriceps and distal medial quadriceps with the patient seated with the knee in approximately 60° of flexion (Fig. 12.3). Suggested parameters are 2500 Hz; 75 bursts/s; 2 s ramp; 10-s on, 50-s rest; intensity to maximum tolerable; 10 contractions per session [6]. Straight leg raises are also a key quadriceps strengthening exercise in this phase. The patient is instructed to dorsiflex the ankle and maintain an isometric quadriceps set (with a visible superior patella glide) before raising the leg to approximately 8 in. Patients work up to three sets of ten repetitions with good form and no extensor lag before resistance is applied.

Weight-bearing exercises are initiated at weeks 3–4 or when the patient is able to perform 50 % weight-bearing on the involved lower extremity. Bilateral calf raises are included to address strengthening of the gastroc–soleus complex.

For patients with a peripheral repair, closed kinetic chain activities will help protect the meniscus and minimize patellar pain [1]. As mentioned earlier, with increasing knee flexion, tensile strain increases across the meniscus. The combination of weight-bearing and knee flexion needs to be balanced during the early rehabilitation phase [3]. End-range knee flexion, as seen in a deep knee bend, generates appreciable shear stress across repair site of longitudinal tears and is usually the mechanism of bucket-handle tear formation [7, 8]. Therefore, deep squats and tibial rotation should be avoided for at least 12 weeks [9].

Phase 2: Early Rehab (Weeks 5–8)

Progression to Phase 2 requires that the patient have minimal knee effusion and pain, in addition to meeting the knee ROM goals, and demonstrate the ability to perform an active straight leg raise without a lag. All Phase 1 exercises will continue as deemed necessary by the physical therapist to meet ROM and strength goals. By the 8-week mark, knee ROM should be full, with manual techniques continuing as needed.

Open kinetic chain strengthening exercises are started at 5–6 weeks postoperatively. Knee extension progressive resistive exercises are limited from 90° to 30° to minimize the patellofemoral joint stress [10]. Closed chain exercises such as mini squats or wall sits (Fig. 12.4) and lateral step-ups are initiated at weeks 7–8, while preventing knee flexion greater than 60° to avoid stressing the repair.

Hamstring strengthening from 0° to 90° can be initiated in patients who had peripheral meniscus repairs between 5 and 6 weeks. For complex repairs, hamstring strengthening can begin at 7 to 8 weeks. Again, care should be taken with isolated resisted hamstring curls due to the semimembranosus insertion along the posteromedial joint capsule as activation may result in traction across a medial repair site. This activity should be progressed with caution and should begin with standing knee flexion without resistance before progressing to ankle cuff weights (Fig. 12.5).

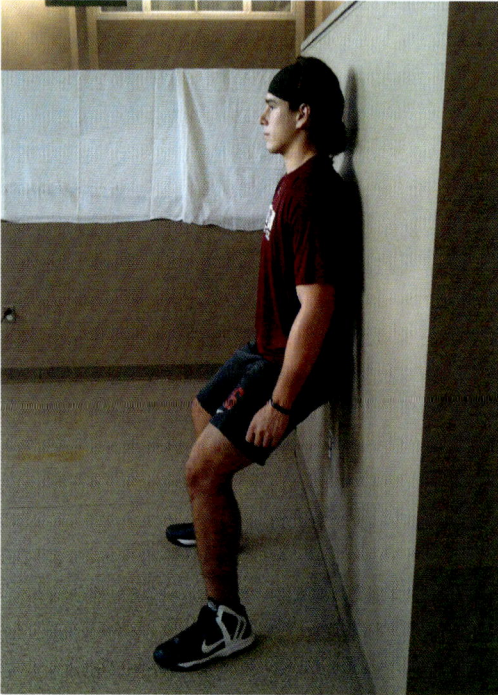

Fig. 12.4 Wall sits are utilized to facilitate quadriceps muscle activation, with the patient limiting the amount of knee flexion to greater than 60° to avoid stressing the repair

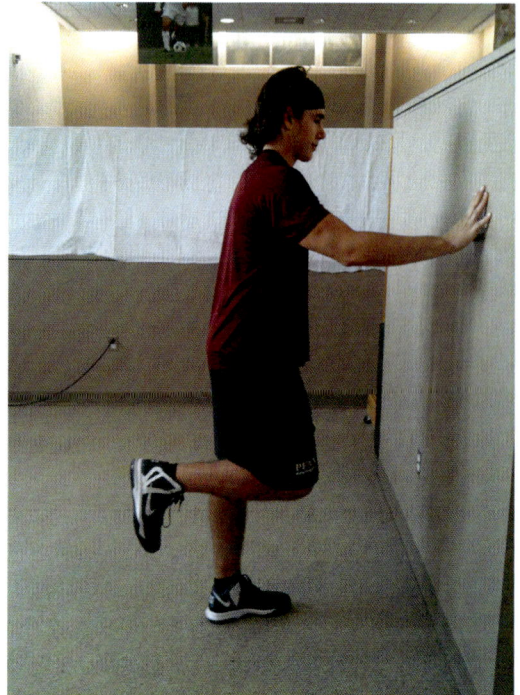

Fig. 12.5 Hamstring strengthening from 0° to 90° is progressed with caution and should begin with standing knee flexion without resistance before progressing to ankle cuff weights. The patient is instructed to maintain a neutral pelvis and hip position

When transitioning to a knee flexion machine in later weeks, the authors recommend utilizing both legs simultaneously to minimize isolated hamstring stress.

Other activities to incorporate at 7–8 weeks include quadriceps and iliotibial band flexibility exercises [1], stationary cycling, and proprioception.

Phase 3: Functional Progression (Weeks 9–12+)

The goals of Phase 3 are to improve strength to the entire lower extremity in addition to enhance proprioception and neuromuscular control of the involved leg. Proximal and core strengthening can be emphasized to provide a stable base for the lower extremity, improve the ability to absorb compressive forces, and maximize lower

extremity function. Knee ROM should be full and with minimal effusion and no pain at this stage. Swimming with flutter kicking can be incorporated to address muscular endurance and conditioning.

Additional closed chain activities that can be progressed in this phase include lunges and sports (resistance) cord activities (Fig. 12.6). It is important to correct form and technique with all exercises, especially closed chain activities where improper mechanics can lead to compensatory movements and elevate the patient's risk for reinjury.

Rehabilitation after meniscal surgery should challenge the balance, stability, and coordination skills of the patient due to the meniscus role in proprioception [11]. Varying body positions (single-limb stance, sport/activity or work specific), varying surfaces (foam, wobble boards, tilt boards, etc.), and varying movement patterns can

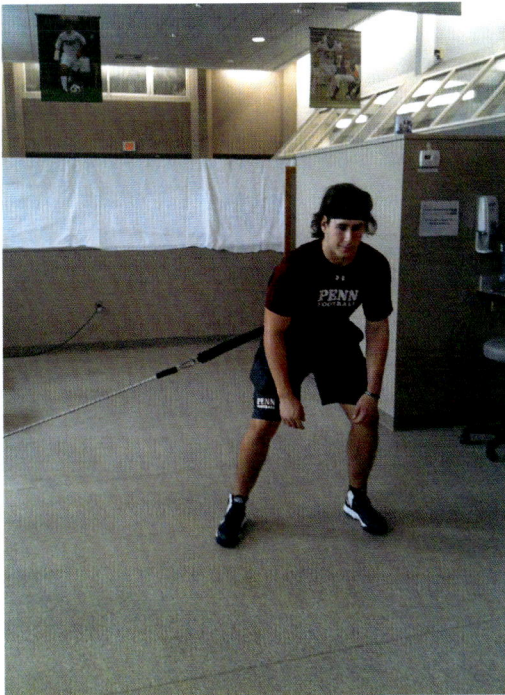

Fig. 12.6 Advanced functional rehabilitation activities can include sports (resistance) cord activities. Variations include lateral stepping (see pic), retro stepping, forward stepping, and multidirectional lunges

be added to the rehabilitation progression of proprioceptive exercises (Fig. 12.7) [12]. Ihara and Nakayama [13] and Wojtys et al. [14] also showed in ACL-deficient patients significantly improved muscle reaction times with proprioceptive and agility training exercises.

Phase 4: Return to Sport/Activity (4 Months+)

The final phase of rehabilitation of meniscal repair is the most important for the athlete working to return to sports. Goals to initiate Phase 4 include full knee ROM, no pain or effusion, satisfactory clinical examination, quadriceps strength of greater than or equal to 75 % versus the contralateral side, hamstrings to quadriceps ratio of greater than or equal to 66 %, and functional hop test(s) of greater than or equal to 70 % versus the

contralateral side. Peripheral tears will be cleared to progress into this phase quicker than patients with a complex tear.

A running program may be initiated at 20 weeks with peripheral meniscus repairs, with complex repairs starting at 30 weeks. Plyometrics are gradually progressed as the patient moved through the first several weeks of the running program. Complex repairs begin plyometrics at 6 months and radial repairs at 9 months. Although very effective at restoring strength and functional status, plyometrics incur the highest strain across repair site and thus are reserved until several months have elapsed. Plyometric training is progressed from double-leg movements to single-leg movements. Additionally, the type of loading can be progressed from medial–lateral to rotational and to deceleration loading (which includes depth work). Heckman et al. [1] advocate plyometrics being incorporated after 6 months postoperatively in patients who have had a large peripheral tear or complex repair and after 9 months postoperatively in patients who had a radial meniscus repair.

Caution should be taken with patients wishing for an early return to strenuous activities, including impact loading, jogging, deep knee flexion, or pivoting. There is a risk of a repeat meniscus tear especially within the first 4–6 months after surgery [2].

Return to Sports

Akin to patients who are returning to sport after ACL reconstruction, functional testing is warranted to clear a patient to both returning to running and retuning to unrestricted sport. Functional testing will allow the clinician to assess how the patient withstands sheer and compressive forces, while evaluating potential biomechanical faults with movement. To this end, hop testing, double-limb and single-limb squatting, and the Star Excursion Balance Test (a dynamic assessment of balance) should be tested prior to initiating a running program and prior to retuning to sport. The single-limb and double-limb squat should be assessed for depth, quality of movement, and the

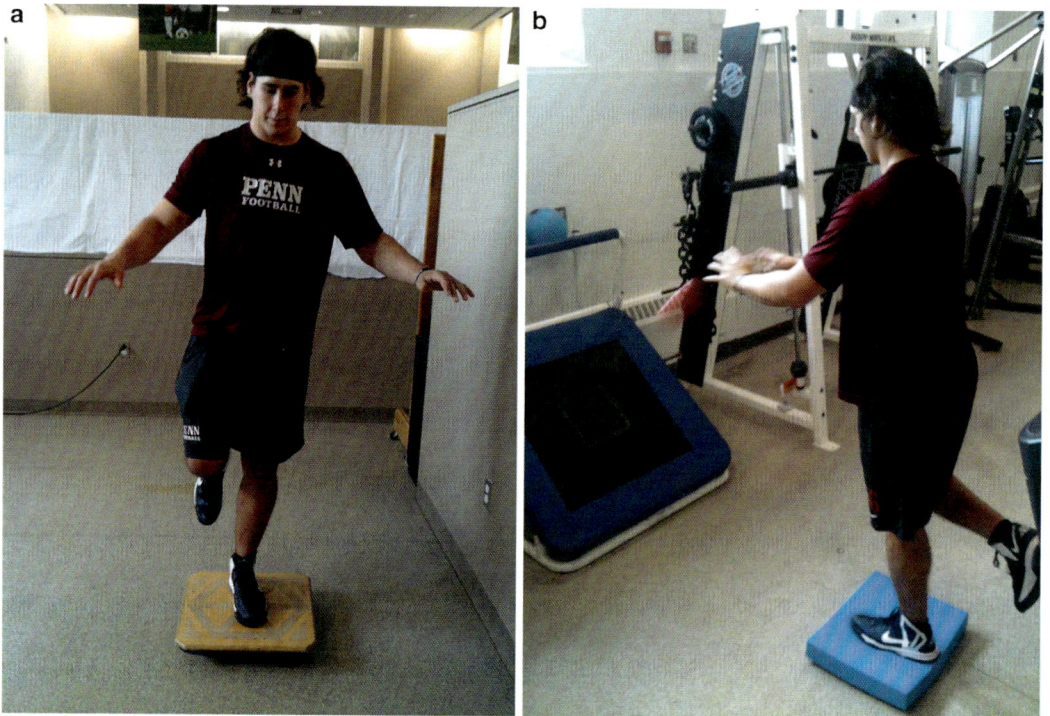

Fig. 12.7 The rehabilitation protocol should include a progression of proprioceptive exercises through varying body positions, surfaces, and movement patterns. Single-limb stance can be progressed to include unstable surfaces such as a tilt board (**a**) and can incorporate dynamic challenges to balance such as a ball toss while maintaining single-limb support (**b**)

presence of pain with movement. Pain during motion or at end range should tell the clinician that impact may not be appropriate at that time. Although biomechanically "at risk" findings such as dynamic valgus are not a contraindication to initiate impact, interventions to correct these faults should be integrated into subsequent sessions.

Typically, a single-limb hop test for distance (Fig. 12.8) is performed prior to initiating a running program. Prior to returning to sport, a hop test battery will provide more comprehensive information as to the patient's readiness to return to unrestricted play, including the single-leg hop for distance, the crossover hop, the triple hop, and the 6-m timed hop test.

Careful biomechanical consideration of the patient's chosen sport or activity should be considered in the later phases of rehabilitation. Aggressive strength, flexibility, agility, power, and speed training may all be components necessary for a patient to regain optimal lower extremity function, and rehabilitation interventions should be specific to mimic the imposed demands of each sport or activity.

Near-perfect limb symmetry should be the goal to return a patient to sport. The patient should demonstrate strength and functional testing of at least 90 % versus the contralateral side; full, symmetrical range of motion; and no pain or difficulty with his or her running program and other sport-specific activities. Graded exercise programs which encompass strength, power, and agility, while mimicking the patient's usual sport or activity as closely as possible, will ultimately return the patient to his or her highest potential functional level.

Red Flags

Progression through the phases of rehabilitation may be hastened or slowed to fit the individual's

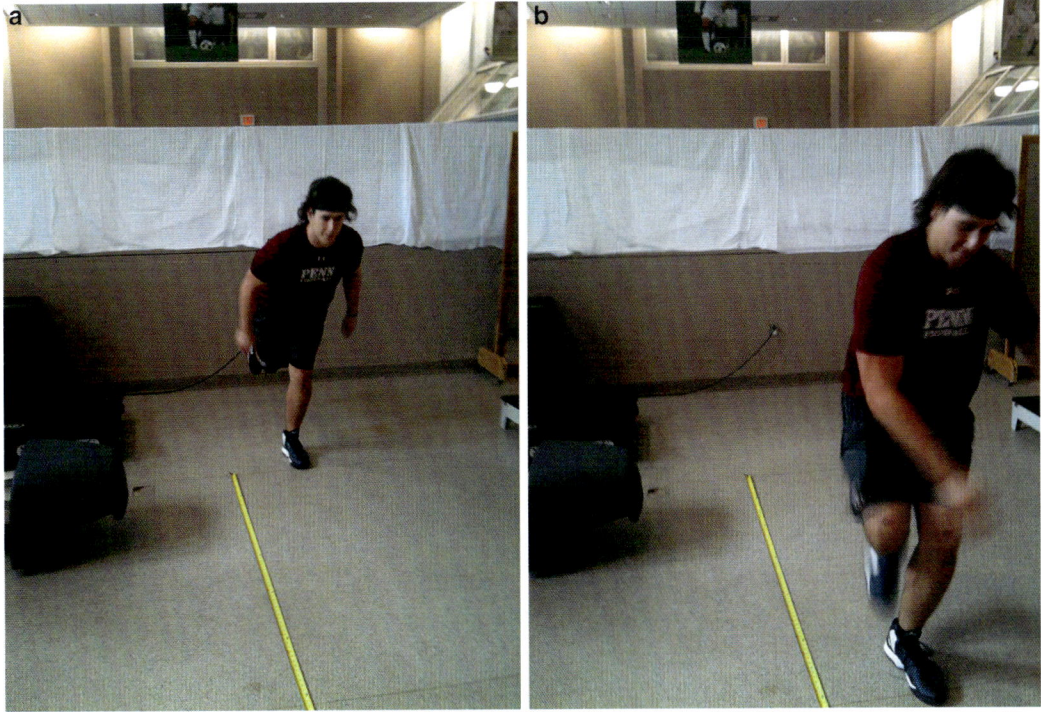

Fig. 12.8 A single-limb hop test for distance is part of a battery of functional hop tests to determine readiness for progression into a running program and/or for return to sport criteria. Patients are instructed to maximally hop from one leg (**a**) and land (**b**) on the same leg without loss of balance. The distance hopped is recorded with difference between the involved and uninvolved legs used to calculate the limb symmetry index. Patients should have normal knee ROM, adequate strength, no pain, no knee joint effusion, good neuromuscular control, and a satisfactory clinical examination prior to progressing to this test

rate of progress, severity of the procedure, and level of activity that the patient is returning to. However, the rehabilitation specialist should be cautious of several "red flags," or warning signs, which warrant contacting the surgeon. Similar to other knee surgeries, calf pain, edema, tenderness, warmth, and diminution of dorsalis pedis pulse may be concern for a deep vein thrombosis. Risk for calf phlebitis is likely higher for "inside out" repairs whereupon a true posterior medial or lateral incision was made. The surgeon should also be contacted if significant joint effusion, warmth, and an unwillingness to bear weight through the involved limb appear. The presence of mechanical symptoms (i.e., catching or locking) may indicate a compromised repair and should be reported to the patient's physician. Failed meniscal repair can be symptomatic or "clinically silent" [15]; however, frequent reevaluation of the patient will caution the clinician to the majority of abnormal findings.

Other Considerations

As previously mentioned, meniscal repairs are often concomitant with other soft tissue, ligamentous, and/or cartilaginous injuries or procedures. Therefore, with rehabilitation procedures, each healing structure should be considered individually to minimize potentially harmful compressive, tensile, or sheer forces. For example, if quadriceps strengthening is desired but the patient has undergone an ACL reconstruction in addition to the meniscal repair, open kinetic chain strengthening should be avoided to reduce the sheer force on the healing ACL. In these cases, the most conservative route should be taken to respect all healing tissues. Furthermore, with locked, bucket-handle tears in an ACL-deficient knee, the surgical intervention may be staged to include a meniscal repair and later an ACL reconstruction after rehabilitation. In this case, the primary goals of rehabilitation are to regain full range of motion, emphasizing extension, and strength within functional limits [15].

Varus and valgus malalignment of the knee may cause increased medial and lateral compartment stress, respectively. These increased stresses may disrupt meniscal healing after repair, so it may be important to consider a knee unloader brace for these patients [3], which functions to reduce the compressive forces sustained by the tibiofemoral joint. Whether or not a patient is braced may be decided by the surgeon's preference.

Conclusion

Rehabilitation following meniscal repair should be individualized based upon the goals of the patient, characteristics of the meniscus tear, and the specifics of the surgical procedure. Patients should be constantly monitored for red flags while providing protection of the healing structures within the appropriate time frames. Communication between the surgeon and physical therapist will help to ensure safe progress through the rehabilitation protocol.

References

1. Heckmann TP, Barber-Westin SD, Noyes FR. Meniscal repair and transplantation: indications, techniques, rehabilitation, and clinical outcome. J Orthop Sports Phys Ther. 2006;36(10):795–814.
2. Noyes FR, Heckmann TP, Barber-Westin SD. Meniscus repair and transplantation: a comprehensive update. J Orthop Sports Phys Ther. 2012;42(3): 274–90.
3. Brotzman SB, Wilk KE. Clinical orthopaedic rehabilitation. 2nd ed. Philadelphia, PA: Mosby; 2003.
4. Barber F, Click S. Meniscal repair rehabilitation with concurrent anterior cruciate reconstruction. J Orthop Sports Phys Ther. 1997;13(4):433–7.
5. Palmieri-Smith RM, Thomas AC, Wojtys EM. Maximizing quadriceps strength after ACL reconstruction. Clin Sports Med. 2008;27(3):405–24.
6. Fitzgerald GK, Piva SR, Irrgang JJ. A modified neuromuscular electrical stimulation protocol for quadriceps strength training following anterior cruciate ligament reconstruction. J Orthop Sports Phys Ther. 2003;33(9):492–501.
7. Becker R, Wirz D, Wolf C, Göpfert B, Nebelung W, Friederich N. Measurement of meniscofemoral contact pressure after repair of bucket-handle tears with biodegradable implants. Arch Orthop Trauma Surg. 2005;125(4):254–60.
8. Johal P, Williams A, Wragg P, Hunt D, Gedroyc W. Tibio-femoral movement in the living knee. A study of weight bearing and non-weight bearing knee kinematics using 'interventional' MRI. J Biomech. 2005; 38(2):269–76.
9. Stärke C, Kopf S, Petersen W, Becker R. Meniscal repair. Arthroscopy. 2009;25(9):1033–44.
10. Steinkamp LA, Dillingham MF, Markel MD, Hill JA, Kaufman KR. Biomechanical considerations in patellofemoral joint rehabilitation. Am J Sports Med. 1993;21(3):438–44.
11. Gray JC. Neural and vascular anatomy of the menisci of the human knee. J Orthop Sports Phys Ther. 1999;29(1):23–30.
12. Bizzini M, Gorelick M, Drobny T. Lateral meniscus repair in a professional ice hockey goaltender: a case report with a 5-year follow-up. J Orthop Sports Phys Ther. 2006;36(2):89–100.
13. Ihara H, Nakayama A. Dynamic joint control training for knee ligament injuries. Am J Sports Med. 1986;14(4):309–15.
14. Wojtys EM, Huston LJ, Taylor PD, Bastian SD. Neuromuscular adaptations in isokinetic, isotonic, and agility training programs. Am J Sports Med. 1996;24(2):187–92.
15. Shelbourne KD, Patel DV, Adsit WS, Porter DA. Rehabilitation after meniscal repair. Clin Sports Med. 1996;15(3):595–612.

Index

Printed by Publishers' Graphics LLC
JCIMO131106.15.17.22